Keto Bread Machine Cookbook

Easy and Delicious Baking Recipes

for Homemade Keto Bread

CONTENTS

INTRODUCTION

This book contains tips and tricks about achieving and maintaining ketosis.

The most critical stage of the ketosis stage is after you achieve it. This book will give you tips and tricks not only about achieving ketosis but maintaining it as well. The book will share techniques on how you can keep the ketosis state wherever you are. Whether you are out dining with friends, on vacation or traveling on business, keeping yourself in ketosis state is possible.

The book also talks about probably one of the largest carbs loaded food, which is bread. Bread, as everyone knows, comes from flour and flour comes from refined grains. The book will give you the answer on how you can eat bread without kicking you out of ketosis. It also includes a brief introduction on bread, bread making and the bread maker machine, plus keto bread recipes you can enjoy for breakfast, lunch and dinner.

Thanks for downloading this book, I hope you enjoy it!

CHAPTER 1

Keto Trips and Tricks

Recently, there's been an influx of interest on Keto Diet and Ketosis. Suddenly, the internet is brimming with information, recipes, and discussions about Keto and Ketosis. Everyone is now looking at what food they are eating and wondering how much of a change Keto would do on their eating habits.

Keto Brief Overview

Keto is short for Ketosis. Ketosis is a normal metabolic process where the body burns stored fats in the absence of enough glucose. When the body does not get enough glucose, stored fats are broken down, and the liver starts to form ketones, which then supplies the body with energy.

However, as the levels of ketones rise, your blood acidity also rises. This could lead to a condition called ketoacidosis. Type 1 diabetics are prone to this condition, which is dangerous because it could lead to coma and death.

When your body starts to burn fats to produce energy, your body is in a Ketogenic stage. To maintain the Ketogenic stage, one must follow the Ketogenic Diet. The Ketogenic Diet or Keto Diet is a diet originally developed to control epilepsy and blood sugar levels of diabetics, and not as a weight loss diet. The diet follows a very low carb, high fat, moderate protein meal plan.

Effective ways to go into Ketosis

So how does one go into Ketosis? Getting your body into Ketogenic stage is not as simple as reducing or eliminating carbs. Here are some helpful tips on how you can effectively get your body into Ketosis:

- **Reduce your carb intake.** Glucose forms a big percentage of carbohydrates and glucose is your main source of energy. Depending on your physical activity and metabolism, not all the glucose in your body burns to produce energy. Excess glucose gets stored in your liver as fatty acids that could lead to damaged liver, kidneys and other internal organs. The level of carbohydrates consumption under Ketosis is individualized but for most, it is between 20 grams to 50 grams net carbs a day. To get the net carb, the equation is total carbohydrates less fiber.

- **Increase your physical activity.** You might say exercise sucks. Exercise doesn't have to be too daunting. You don't have to go to the gym or take exercise classes. You can do something as simple as walking. If you are walking 5 minutes a day, increase that to 15 to 30 minutes a day. You can go up a flight of stairs instead of using an elevator to get 3 to 5 stores high. The bottom line is moving your body.

- **Increase fat intake.** Fat here refers to healthy fats like unsaturated fats. Avoid saturated fats and trans fats that can raise bad cholesterol levels. To help boost ketones production, your body needs to consume 60% of your calorie intake from fat.

- **Consume enough protein.** The original ketogenic diet used in epilepsy restricts carb and protein to get maximum ketone levels. But for majority of people, cutting down on protein is not healthy. Protein supplies the liver with amino acids to make new glucose. It also helps maintain muscle mass when you cut down on carbs. Adequate protein intake should range from 0.55 grams to 0.77 grams per pound of lean mass.

- **Add coconut oil in your diet.** Coconut oil contains fats called MCT or medium-chain triglycerides. MCT is absorbed and taken directly to the liver compared to other fats, allowing your body to immediately turn MCT into energy or convert it into ketones. A word of caution though, when consuming coconut oil, try to do it slowly to lessen digestive effects like diarrhea and stomach cramps.

- **Replenish your body with water.** Achieving ketosis is not possible if you are dehydrated. Cutting down on carbs will cut down your water and sodium intake. Add a pinch of salt on your water to replenish the salt you are losing from cutting down on carbs.

- **Track your ketone levels.** There is no benchmark to know if you are in ketosis. This is why tracking your ketone levels is important. There are three ways you can test ketone levels. One is through breath, another is by blood, and the last is by urine. Using any of these methods will help you gauge how much adjustments you need make to achieve and maintain ketosis. You are in ketosis if your ketone level reaches 0.8 millimoles per liter.

Getting into Keto in 24 hours

In today's modern world, everyone wants everything done yesterday. People want instant gratification, and 2 to 4 days to get into ketosis state is not acceptable for them. They want immediate results and if they can do it in one day or less, the better. But, can you achieve ketosis in 24 hours? The answer is yes, it is possible. Just follow these simple tips:

- **Do 24-hour fasting or intermittent fasting.** Fasting creates a wide gap between meals, forcing your body to survive without the carbs. If your body cannot find the glucose, it will start to break the fats to produce ketones and burn it to produce energy.

- **Hydrate and stock up on minerals and electrolytes.** This will help you fight against the keto flu. There are available electrolytes in the market. You can also buy magnesium and potassium supplements or make a DIY electrolyte drink by mixing a cup of water, a pinch of salt and 2 tablespoons of lemon juice. Drink plenty of water with a pinch of salt to hydrate and replenish sodium.

- **If you are doing intermittent fasting, eat leafy greens like spinach and kale, nuts, and seeds.** Do not eat food rich in sugar and carbohydrates. Eat nutritious foods.

- **Take supplements that would boost your ketone levels.** There are supplements available in the market to help increase your ketone levels. It is advisable to check with your doctor before taking any ketone supplement because too much ketones can lead to adverse effects.

Keto Diet Tips for Beginners

Once you achieve ketosis, the biggest hurdle you are going to face is maintaining it. The first few weeks are the most critical phase when your body tries to adapt to the changes, and it is a big change. Your body is used to running on glucose for energy and suddenly, you switch to using fats to produce energy. Your body will be resistant to the change, and if you cannot get your body to adapt to these changes, you will have a hard time maintaining the ketosis state.

Here are some neat tricks that you can do to help your body adjust while you are in keto-adaption:

- The level of carb consumption under keto is individualized so you need to find out what should be your macronutrient breakdown. Do not adhere to the standard 20 grams per day minimum carb intake. Instead, check what amount of carbs, protein and fat your body needs.

- Set a goal why you are going into ketosis. This makes it easier to maintain the diet. If you are suffering from diabetes, it is best to consult your doctor first. Rapid change in your sugar level can lead to dizziness and severe sugar withdrawal.

- Learn to read nutrition labels of food. If the food has no label like fresh food, you can search the internet for the nutrition info. Avoid foods with added sugar.

- Always keep low carb snacks handy. You can prepare DIY easy keto snacks like mix almonds and walnuts or keto crackers.

- Always keep yourself hydrated. Keep a bottle of water in your bag or if you have time, prepare a hand carry tumbler of electrolyte drink (mix of water, fresh lemon juice and salt).

- If you are not eating out, prepare homemade keto recipes and bring at work, or when you travel.

Eating Out while on Keto

Cooking your own food is the best way to ensure that what you are eating will not kick you out of ketosis. However, there will be days when you have to eat out with friends, or have a lunch meeting with clients, or just simply want to eat out in a restaurant. If you are on Keto Diet, this could pose a big problem.

If you must eat out, here are some tips you can follow:

- **Make your plans.** When you eat out, you don't normally decide on it out of the blue. If you know where you are going to eat, you can call the restaurant in advance and check if you can adjust with your meals. You can also find keto-friendly restaurants and suggest it to your friends or clients.

- **Choose your food and substitute.** If you cannot avoid non-keto restaurants, then try to order food that is rich in healthy fat, with moderate protein and low carb. If the restaurant is offering steaks and fries, substitute the fries with steamed veggies or order a veggie salad. If you cannot substitute, then don't eat the fries.

- **Watch out for the condiments and dressings.** If you order a salad, make sure the dressing is keto-friendly. Most spices are keto-friendly. Even if it says vinaigrette dressing, it won't hurt to ask and confirm. You never know if it includes hidden ingredients.

- **Choose your beverages.** If you are eating out, stick with water, water with lemon, soda water, unsweetened tea and black coffee. Try to avoid alcohol. If you cannot avoid it, choose a glass of dry white or red wine. If you prefer hard alcohol, go for vodka, gin, whiskey, dry martini or brandy, which are low carb.

- **Do not hesitate to ask questions.** If you have no control over choosing the restaurant and unable to call ahead, raise questions. It may annoy the waiter but ensuring that you don't accidentally eat food that will kick you out of keto is more important.

- **Order dessert substitute.** Most restaurants won't carry keto-friendly desserts. If you know what food you should eat, you will be able to substitute a blueberry cheesecake with berries in heavy cream or order dark chocolate. There is also the option of skipping dessert.

Travelling on Vacation while on Keto

Travelling has always been in everyone's bucket list. Whether you are going with your partner, family, or even just a business trip, going to a new place is always exciting and fun. Unfortunately, with travelling also comes the problem of where you are going to eat if you are on a strict diet, especially a Keto Diet.

Below are some neat tips if you are travelling or planning a vacation:

- Search for keto-friendly restaurants in the area where you plan to travel. Read testimonials from visitors to know if they are keto-friendly.

- Find out if you can prepare or cook your own meals where you plan to stay.

- If you cannot cook, prepare meals that only requires preparation like salads and sandwiches.

- Pack low carb food when you travel.

Staying in Keto is a matter of discipline and does not depend on where you eat.

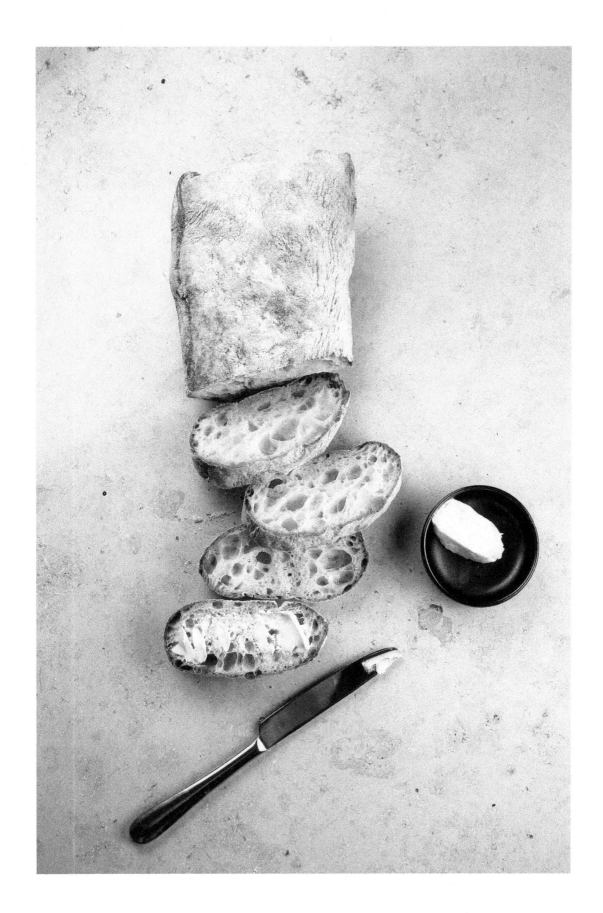

CHAPTER 2

Eating Bread While on Keto

A staple food is a food regularly eaten in quantities that make it predominantly standard diet for some people. Some common staple foods include meat, eggs, fish, cheese, root vegetables or tubers like potatoes and cassava, starchy tubers, and cereals from which bread is made.

Different Types of Bread

There are many types of bread, but there are three categories to which the many types of bread can be classified into. The first are breads that rise high and have to be baked in pans like bread loaves and muffins; the second are breads with medium volume like baguettes, rye bread, and other French bread; and the last are those that hardly rise or more known as flatbread like naan bread, tortilla bread, pizza bread, and crackers.

Some of the most popular breads that people normally eat for breakfast, lunch or dinner include:

- Loaves. These are rounded or oblong mass of dough baked in rectangular pans. Loaves come in white bread, multi-grain, brown bread, Ezekiel bread and many others. The loaves are the most common type of bread.

- Bagels. Bagel is a type of bread resembling a doughnut but unlike regular bread, bagels are prepared by boiling first in water before baking.

- Pizza. Pizza is a round flatbread topped by tomato sauce, cheese and some added meat and vegetables. The pizza is of Italian origin. Pizza can also be prepared using a loaf bread.

- Muffins. Muffins are prepared and baked like cakes, but muffins are a type of bread and not cake. Muffins are usually eaten for breakfast and can be sweet or savory.

- Breadsticks. Breadstick is a dry bread that resembles thin-sized pencils in form and normally used as a dipping stick. Breadstick originated from Turin, Italy, and is usually served as an appetizer.

- Crackers. Cracker is a type of bread made from wheat flour and water and comes in many forms like rye and multi-grain.

Basic Steps to Make Bread

Bread is usually prepared from combining flour and water to form a dough and commonly cooked by baking. Bread has played a significant role in the history of man-made food throughout the world.

Below is a basic guide on how to make bread:

- Scaling refers to measuring of ingredients and the most important in the bread making process. A slight change in the measurement can affect how your bread will turn out.

- Mix all ingredients you measure to prepare it for fermentation and development of gluten. The key to mixing is time and speed.

- Next is allowing the dough to rise or the fermentation process. During this time, the yeast converts the dough's natural sugars into carbon dioxide and ethanol. The carbon dioxide is what makes the dough rise.

- After fermentation, you need to release some of the trapped carbon dioxide in the gluten. This is the punching or degassing process. This process also helps the gluten to relax, distribute the nutrients, and equalize the temperature of the dough inside and out.

- Next process is cutting or dividing. Dividing the dough will help you easily manage the dough during the next stages. You can cut and weigh the dough into smaller sizes.

- The next step is shaping your dough to your desired type of bread. You can shape it into a loaf, a ball, or a long torpedo.

- Next is resting or benching. You set aside your pre-shaped dough to rest and make the gluten relax. Resting time varies from a few minutes or more.

- Next process is the final shaping and panning. After resting, you can knead the dough and get it into its final shape. You can shape it into a ball, baguette, torpedo, braid, or loaf before putting it in the baking pan.

- Most breads with yeast undergo two fermentation. The first one is bulk fermentation and the second is during proofing. During proofing, the dough can rise to its baking size.

- After proofing, the bread is ready to go into the oven to bake.

- Once baked, the bread goes on cooling racks to cool down.

- Last step is storing and packing of the bread.

How Do Bread Making Machines Work?

The best thing about using a bread-making machine is it gets the hard cycle of bread making easy. You can use the bread-making machine in complete cycle, especially for loaf bread or you can just do the dough cycle if you are baking bread that needs to bake in an oven. To use the bread-making machine, here are some steps to guide you:

- **Familiarize yourself with the parts and buttons of your bread-making machine.**

  Your bread-making machine has three important parts and without it, you will not be able to cook your bread. The first part is the machine itself, second is the bread bucket and the third is the kneading blade. The bread bucket and kneading blade are removable and replaceable. You can check with the manufacturer for parts to replace it if it's missing.

  Learn how to operate your bread-making machine. Removing and placing the bread bucket back in is important. Practice snapping the bread bucket on and off the machine until you are comfortable doing it. This is important because you don't want the bucket moving once the ingredients are in place.

- **Know your bread bucket capacity.**

This is an important step before you start using the machine. If you load an incorrect measurement, you are going to have a big mess on your hand. To check your bread bucket capacity:

- o Use a liquid measuring cup and fill it with water.

- o Pour the water on the bread bucket until it's full. Count how many cups of water you poured on the bread bucket.

- o The number of cups of water will determine the size of your loaf bread.

Less than 10 cups	=	1-pound loaf
10 cups	=	1 to 1 ½ pounds loaf
12 cups	=	1 or 1 ½ to 2 pounds loaf
14 cups or more	=	1 or ½ to 2 or 2 ½ pounds loaf

- **Learn the basic buttons and settings of your bread-making machine.**

  Here are some tips you can do to familiarize yourself with the machine:

  o Read all the button labels. The buttons indicate the cycle in which your machine will mix, knead, and bake the bread.

  o Basic buttons include START/STOP, CRUST COLOR, TIMER/ARROW, SELECT (BASIC, SWEET, WHOLE WHEAT, FRENCH, GLUTEN FREE, QUICK/RAPID, QUICK BREAD, JAM, DOUGH.)

  o The SELECT button allows you to choose the cycle you want in which you want to cook your loaf. It also includes DOUGH cycle for oven-cooked breads.

Using the Delay button.

When you select a cycle, the machine sets a preset timer to bake the bread. Example, if you select BASIC, time will be set by 3 hours. However, you want your bread cooked at a specific time, say, you want it at 12 noon but it's only 7:00 in the morning. Your bread cooks for 3 hours, which means it will be done by 10:00 am but you want it done by 12. You can use the up and down arrow key to set the delay timer. Between 7 am and 12 noon, there is a difference of 5 hours so you want your timer to be set at 5. Press the arrow keys up to add 2 hours in your timer so that your bread will cook in 5 hours instead of 3 hours. Delay button does not work if you are using the DOUGH cycle.

- **Order of adding the ingredients**

This only matters if you are using the delay timer. It is important to ensure that your yeast will not touch any liquid so as not to activate it early. Early activation of the yeast could make your bread rise too much. If you plan to start the cycle immediately, you can add the ingredients in any order. However, adding the ingredients in order will discipline you to do it every time and make you less likely to forget it when necessary. To add the ingredients, do it in the following order:

- o First, place all the liquid ingredients in the bread bucket.

- o Add the sugar and the salt.

- o Add the flour to cover and seal in the liquid ingredients.

- o Add all the other remaining dry ingredients.

- o Lastly, add the yeast. The yeast should not touch any liquid until the cooking cycle starts. When adding the yeast, make a small well using your finger to place the yeast to ensure proper timing of yeast activation.

Using the Dough Cycle

You cannot cook all breads using the bread-making machine, but you can use the machine to make the bread-making process easier. All bread goes under the dough cycle. If your bread needs to be oven-cooked, you can still use the bread-making machine by selecting the DOUGH cycle to mix and knead your flour into a dough. To start the Dough cycle:

- Add all your bread recipe ingredients in your bread bucket.

- Select the DOUGH cycle. This takes usually between 40 to 90 minutes.

- Press the START button.

- After the cycle is complete, let your dough rest in the bread-making machine for 5 to 40 minutes.

- Take out the dough and start cutting into your desire shape.

Some machines have Pasta Dough or Cookie Dough cycle, which you can use for muffin recipes. However, if all you have is basic dough setting, you can use it for muffin recipe, but you need to stop the machine before the rising cycle begins.

What Is Keto Bread?

As a staple food, bread is part of your everyday meal plan even if you are in ketosis. However, flour and sugar as its main ingredient makes bread one of your number one enemy if you are in a keto diet. This does not mean though that you cannot have bread in your keto diet meal plan.

You can still eat any kind of bread by substituting flour with keto friendly alternatives like almond flour and coconut flour as shown in the sample recipes you will find in this book. All the bread recipes were prepared using the bread-making machine and cooked in bread-maker or the oven.

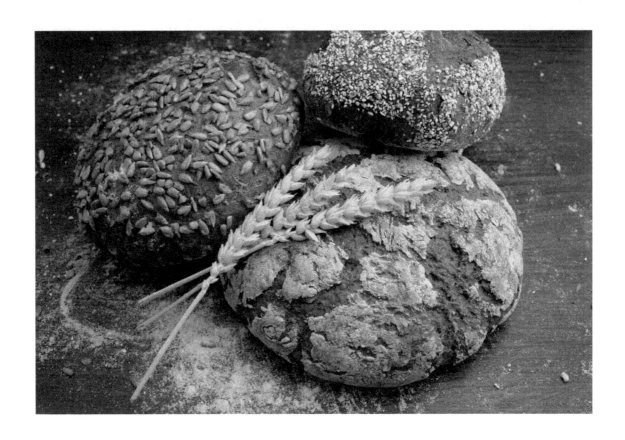

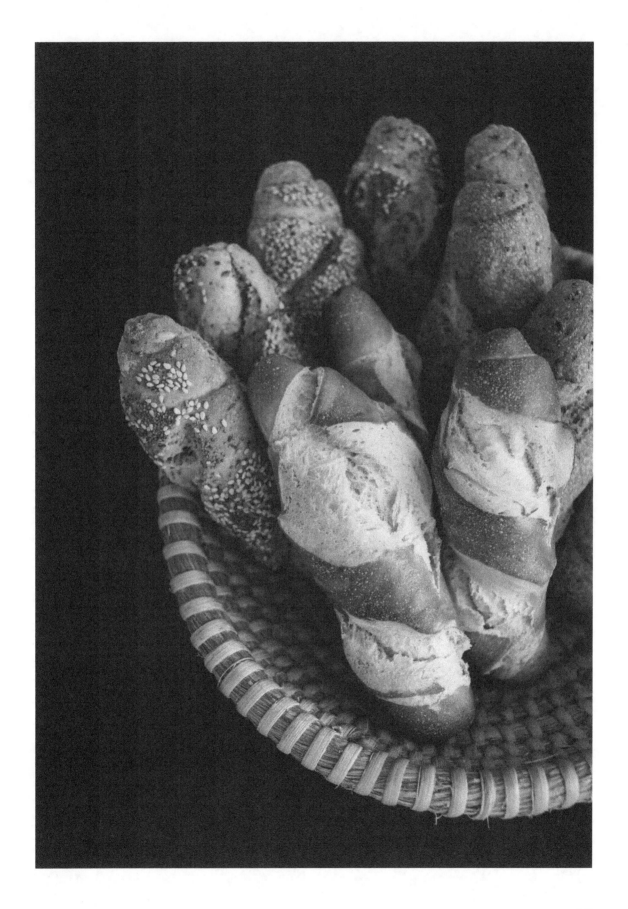

CHAPTER 3

Keto Bread Recipes for Breakfast

Breakfast is the most important meal of the day and having a nutritious food packed with vitamins, minerals and protein will help jumpstart your day. Try these delicious bread recipes to fill you up before your next meal.

Keto Yeast Loaf Bread

Nutrition Facts

Calories: 99

Calories from fat: 45

Total Fat: 5 g

Total Carbohydrates: 7 g

Net Carbohydrates: 5 g

Protein: 9 g

Preparation + Cook Time

Preparation Time: 5 minutes

Cooking Time: 4 hours

Total Time: 4 hours 5 minutes

Servings

16 slices (1 slice per serving)

Ingredients

- 1 package dry yeast (rapid rise or highly active)

- ½ tsp. sugar (real sugar)

- 1 1/8 cup warm water about 90-100 degrees F

- 3 tbsps. Olive oil or avocado oil

- 1 cup vital wheat gluten flour

- ¼ cup oat flour

- ¾ cup soy flour

- ¼ cup flax meal

- ¼ cup wheat bran course, unprocessed

- 1 tbsp. sugar (real sugar)

- 1 ½ tsp. baking powder

- 1 tsp. salt

Directions

- Mix the sugar, water and yeast in the bread bucket to proof the yeast. If the yeast does not bubble, toss and replace it.

- Combine all the dry ingredients in a bowl and mix thoroughly. Pour over the wet ingredients in the bread bucket.

- Set the bread machine and select BASIC cycle to bake the loaf. Close the lid. This takes 3 to 4 hours.

- When the cycle ends, remove the bread from the bread machine.

- Cool on a rack before slicing.

- Serve with butter or light jam.

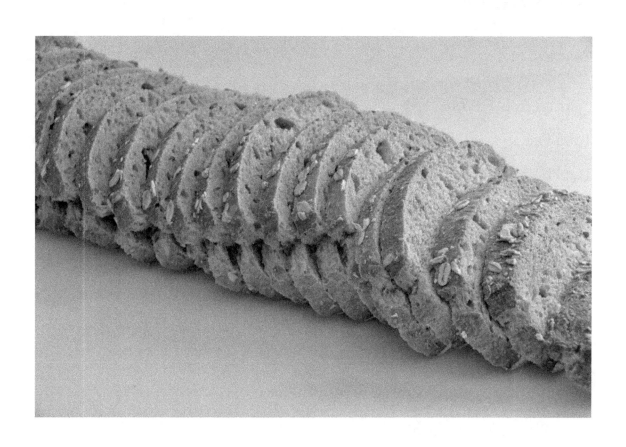

Keto Banana Almond Bread

Nutrition Facts

Calories: 147

Calories from fat: 90

Total Fat: 10 g

Total Carbohydrates: 13 g

Net Carbohydrates: 12 g

Protein: 2 g

Preparation + Cook Time

Preparation Time: 20 minutes

Cooking Time: 2 hours

Total Time: 2 hours 20 minutes

Servings

12 slices

Ingredients

- 2 large eggs

- 1/3 cup butter, unsalted

- 1/8 cup almond milk, unsweetened

- 2 medium mashed bananas

- 1 1/3 cup almond flour

- 0.63 tsp. Stevia extract sugar

- 1 ¼ tsps. Baking powder

- ½ tsp. baking soda

- ½ tsp. salt

- ½ cup chopped nuts

Directions

- Prepare all the ingredients.

- Ensure all ingredients are at room temperature. Place the butter, eggs, milk, and mashed bananas in the bread bucket.

- In a mixing bowl, combine all the dry ingredients and mix well.

- Pour the dry ingredients in the bread bucket.

- Set the bread machine in QUICK BREAD then close the lid and let it cook until the machine beeps.

- Cool the bread before slicing and serving.

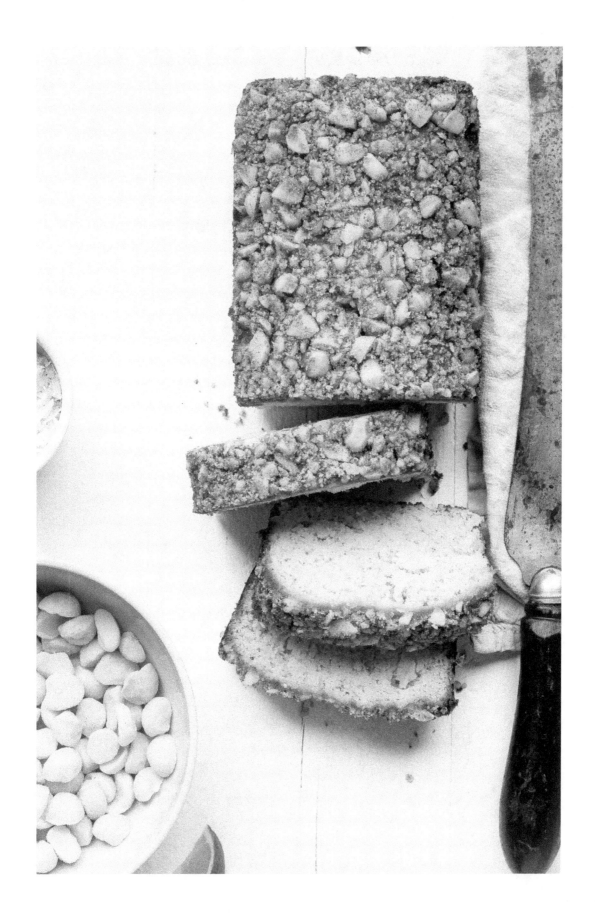

Keto Blueberry-Banana Loaf

Nutrition Facts

Calories: 119

Calories from fat: 90

Total Fat: 9 g

Total Carbohydrates: 9 g

Net Carbohydrates: 7 g

Protein: 2 g

Preparation + Cook Time

Preparation Time: 10 minutes

Cooking Time: 2 hours 20 minutes

Total Time: 2 hours 30 minutes

Servings

12 slices

Ingredients

- ½ cup warm water

- 1 tbsp. almond milk, unsweetened

- 2 eggs, small

- 8 tbsps. Butter, melted and unsalted

- 3 medium sized mashed bananas

- 0.75 tsp. stevia extract

- 2 cups almond flour

- ½ tsp. salt

- 2 tsps. Baking powder

- 1 tsp. baking soda

- 1 cup frozen blueberries

Directions

- Prepare the ingredients. Beat the eggs and mash the bananas. Soften the butter in the microwave for 30 seconds. Mix the water and the milk.

- Put the bananas, eggs, butter, water and milk in the bread bucket.

- Add in all the dry ingredients except blueberries.

- Start the bread machine by selecting QUICK BREAD then close the lid. After the first kneading, open the lid and add in the blueberries. Close the lid and let the cycle continue until the end.

- Once cooked, remove the bread from the bucket and let it cool in a cooling rack before slicing.

- Serve.

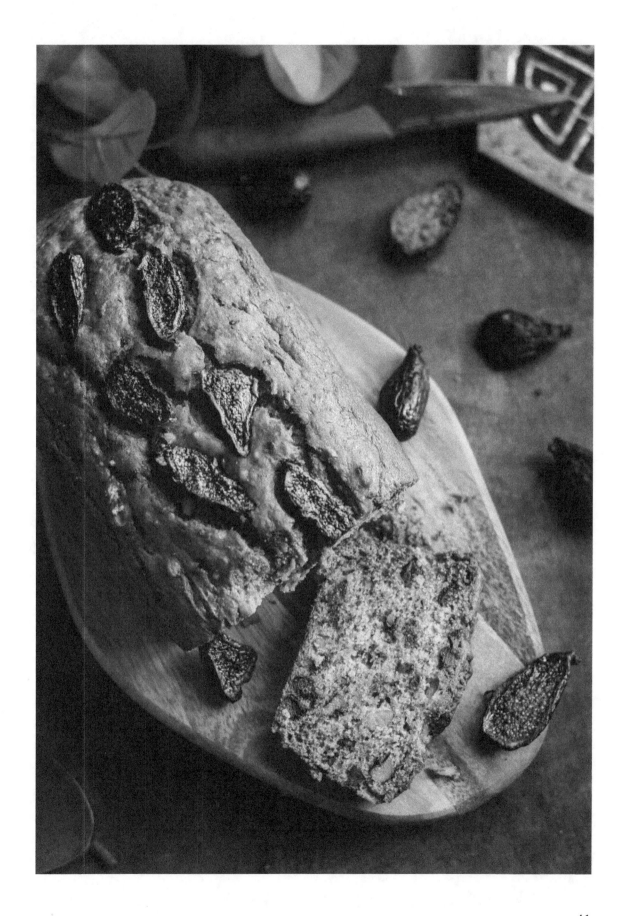

Keto Breakfast Meat Lovers Pizza

Nutrition Facts

Calories: 470

Calories from fat: 333

Total Fat: 37 g

Total Carbohydrates: 4 g

Net Carbohydrates: 3 g

Protein: 28 g

Preparation + Cook Time

Preparation Time: 90 minutes

Cooking Time: 30 minutes

Total Time: 2 hours

Servings

8 slices

Ingredients

Crust

- 2 cups mozzarella cheese, shredded

- 2 tbsps. Cream cheese

- 1 egg

- ¾ cup almond flour

Toppings

- 6 eggs

- 2 tbsps. Heavy cream

- 1 tbsp. butter

- ½ cup crumbled bacon

- ½ cup cooked crumbled breakfast sausage

- ½ cup cheese sauce

- ¼ cup cheddar, shredded

- 2 tbsps. Green onions, chopped

Cheese Sauce

- 1 ¼ cup heavy whipping cream

- 2 oz. cream cheese

- 2 tbsps. Butter

- ½ tsp. ground mustard

- ½ tsp. pepper

- 6 oz. grated cheddar

- 3 oz. grated gruyere

Directions

- To start the crust, combine and melt the mozzarella and cream cheese in the microwave for 30 seconds.

- Pour the cheese melt in the bread bucket then add the eggs and almond flour. Place the bread bucket inside the bread machine.

- Turn the bread machine on by selecting DOUGH cycle, close the lid then press start and wait for the cycle to finish in about 90 minutes.

- While waiting for the dough, prepare the cheese sauce by combining whip cream, cream cheese, and butter in a saucepan over medium heat until melted.

- Whisk in the mustard and pepper.

- Remove from heat and whisk in the cheddar and gruyere until it turns creamy.

- Preheat your oven at 425 degrees F before you start shaping the dough. Prepare a pizza pan and spray with non-stick baking spray. Set aside.

- Roll your dough into a 12-inch diameter circle between 2 sheets of parchment paper.

- Bake for 10 minutes until golden brown.

- To do the sauce and toppings, whisk six eggs and cream in a bowl until combined.

- Heat butter over medium fire in a large skillet. Add the egg mixture and scramble the egg until it turns soft fluffy and slightly wet appearance.

- Spread ½ cup of the cheese sauce onto the pizza crust, then topped with the scrambled egg, bacon, and sausage. Sprinkle the grated cheddar on top.

- Return to the over for another 5 minutes.

- Remove from the oven and sprinkle green onions on top.

- Slice and serve.

Notes:

Cheese sauce recipe yields 2 ½ cups and you only need ½ cup for the pizza. You can store the remaining sauce in an air tight lidded jar.

Recipe nutrition info includes the ½-cup cheese sauce.

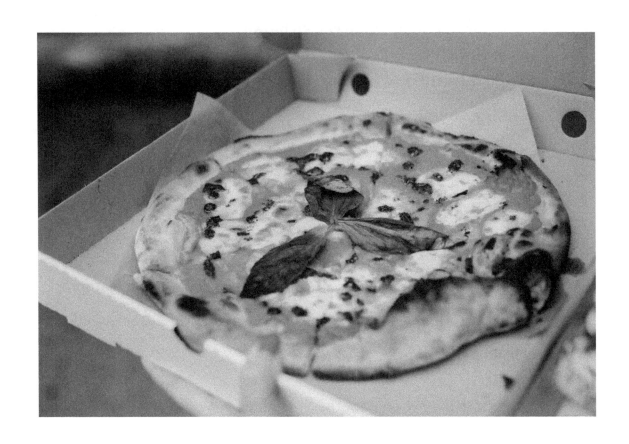

Keto English Muffin Loaf

Nutrition Facts

Calories: 22

Calories from fat: 9

Total Fat: 1 g

Total Carbohydrates: 3 g

Net Carbohydrates: 3 g

Protein: 2 g

Preparation + Cook Time

Preparation Time: 10 minutes

Cooking Time: 3 hours

Total Time: 3 hours 10 minutes

Servings

1-pound loaf of 8 slices (1 slice per serving)

Ingredients

- 1 cup warm water (80 degrees F)

- 2 tbsps. Sugar

- 3 tbsps. Non-fat dry milk

- 1 tsp. salt

- ¼ tsp baking soda

- 2 ½ cups almond flour

- 1 tbsp. vital wheat gluten

- 1 ¾ tsp. dry active yeast

Directions

- Measure all the ingredients in the bread machine pan in the order listed above.

- Turn on bread machine and process. Select BASIC cycle; choose normal CRUST COLOR setting. Close the lid and press START button.

- Once cooked, place bread in cooling rack.

- Slice, then toast and serve.

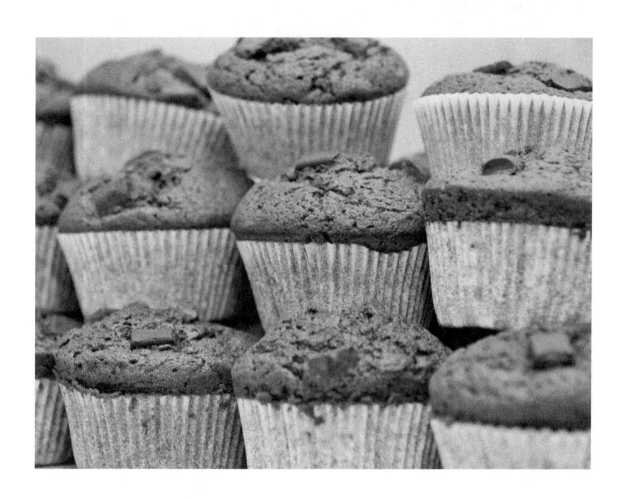

Keto Ciabatta Bread

Nutrition Facts

Calories: 286

Calories from fat: 171

Total Fat: 19 g

Total Carbohydrates: 9 g

Net Carbohydrates: 5 g

Protein: 21

Preparation + Cook Time

Preparation Time: 120 minutes

Cooking Time: 40 minutes

Total Time: 2 hours 40 minutes

Servings

6 slices (1/3 of a loaf per slice)

Ingredients

- 1 cup + 2 tbsps. warm water, divided

- 1 tsp. sugar

- 2 ¼ tsp. dry active yeast

- 1 cup vital wheat gluten

- 1 cup super fine almond flour

- ¼ cup flax seed meal

- ¾ tsp. salt

- 1 ½ tsp. baking powder

- 3 tbsps. extra virgin olive oil

- 1 tbsp. melted butter

Directions

- In a bowl, combine ½-cup warm water, sugar and yeast. Cover and let it sit for 10 minutes or until frothy.

- In your bread machine bucket, add the yeast mixture, the remaining ½ cup and 2 tbsps. water, and olive oil. Add flour, flax seed, salt, and baking powder. Place the bread bucket back in the bread machine and close the lid.

- Set the bread machine to DOUGH cycle, close the lid then press the START button. After 10 minutes, stop the bread machine. You will have a very sticky dough.

- Pour the dough on a floured surface and divide into half before rolling into tube like shape (about 2.5 x 7 inches). Place the cut dough on a greased cookie sheet.

- Preheat your oven for 2 to 3 minutes at 110 degrees F. Turn the oven off and place the dough inside to rise for 1 hour. After 1 hour, you should have about 3.5 x 8 inches raised dough.

- Preheat your oven at 350 degrees F to start baking.

- Brush your raised dough with melted butter, then bake for 15 minutes. Take out of the oven and brush once more with butter before returning inside the oven for another 10 to 15 minutes until the dough's internal temperature reaches 200 degrees F.

- Once done, let the loaf cool for 1 hour before slicing.

- Serve with scrambled egg or your favorite jam.

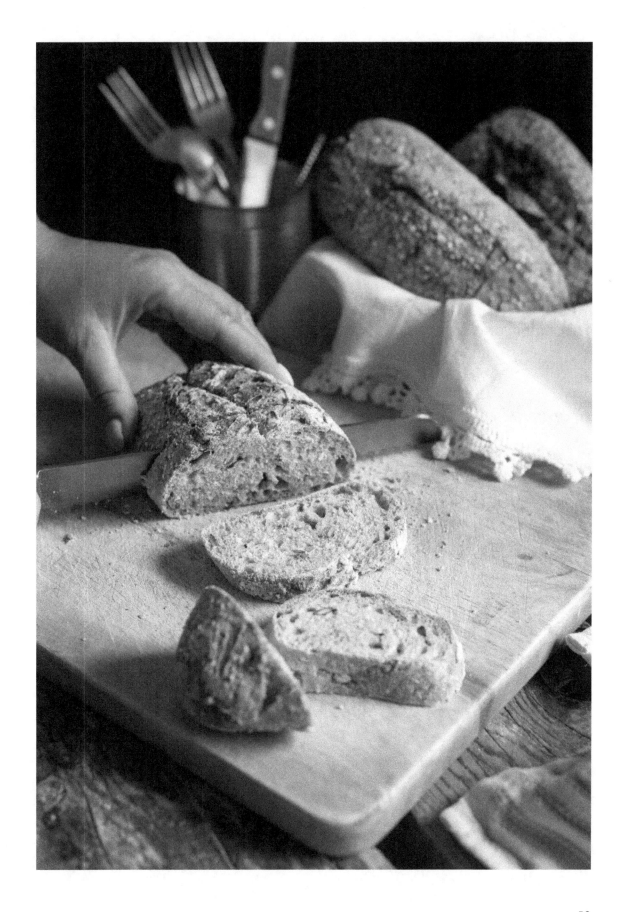

Keto Almond Cinnamon Rolls

Nutrition Facts

Calories: 124

Calories from fat: 100

Total Fat: 11 g

Total Carbohydrates: 8 g

Net Carbohydrates: 7 g

Protein: 2 g

Preparation + Cook Time

Preparation Time: 2 hours 35 minutes

Cooking Time: 20 minutes

Total Time: 2 hours 55 minutes

Servings

12 rolls

Ingredients

- 1 cup almond milk, unsweetened

- 1 large egg

- 4 tbsps. butter

- 3 1/3 cup almond flour

- 3 tbsps. sugar

- ½ tsp. salt

- 2 tsps. dry active yeast

Cinnamon Filling

- ¼ cup melted butter

- ¼ cup swerve sweetener

- 2 tsps. cinnamon powder

- ½ tsp. nutmeg

- 1/3 cup dry roasted mixed nuts

Directions

- Add all the ingredients of the cinnamon bread in the bread bucket according to the order of appearance in the ingredients list.

- On your bread machine, select DOUGH cycle, close the lid then press START and let the machine do its work.

- Once cycle is finished, take out the dough and knead the dough on a floured surface for a minute. Let it rest for 15 minutes.

- Preheat your oven at 375 degrees F. Prepare a greased 13 x 9-inch baking pan and set aside.

- Roll the dough into 15 x 10-inch rectangle. Spread ¼ cup of melted butter over the dough about one inch from the edges.

- Sprinkle the sugar, nutmeg, cinnamon and mixed nuts over the dough evenly. Roll the dough tightly from one edge then press to seal, forming a 12-inch long roll.

- Cut the dough into one-inch size and arrange on the greased baking pan. Cover and let it rise for 30 to 45 minutes.

- Put it in the oven. Allow to bake for 20 to 25 minutes or until it turns golden brown.

- Cool for about 10-15 minutes.

- You have the option to serve with powdered sugar icing or serve warm as is.

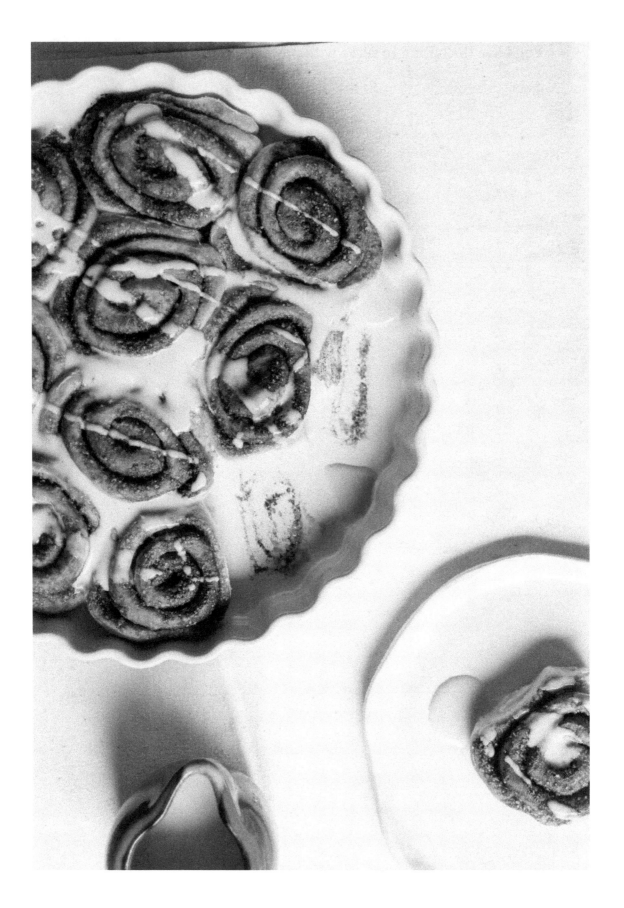

Keto Kalamata Olive Loaf

Nutrition Facts

Calories: 161

Calories from fat: 130

Total Fat: 14 g

Total Carbohydrates: 8 g

Net Carbohydrates: 5 g

Protein: 5 g

Preparation + Cook Time

Preparation Time: 2 hours

Cooking Time: 10 minutes

Total Time: 2 hours 10 minutes

Servings

10 slices

Ingredients

- ½ cup brine from olives

- 1 cup warm water

- 2 tbsps. olive oil

- 1 ½ tsp. salt

- 2 tbsps. sugar

- 3 cups almond flour

- 1 2/3 cup almond meal

- 1 ½ tsp. dried basil leaves

- 2 tsps. active dry yeast

- ½ cup olives finely chopped

Directions

- Combine the brine and warm water.

- Using the bread bucket, put all ingredients except olives in the order of their appearance on the ingredient list starting with the brine mixture.

- Select the WHEAT BREAD cycle on your machine. If there is no WHEAT BREAD cycle, you can select BASIC cycle. Close the cover and press START.

- With the first beep of the machine, open the lid and add in the olives. Close the lid and let the cycle continue.

- When the cycle ends, you can take the loaf out and let it cool in a cooling rack.

- Slice before serving.

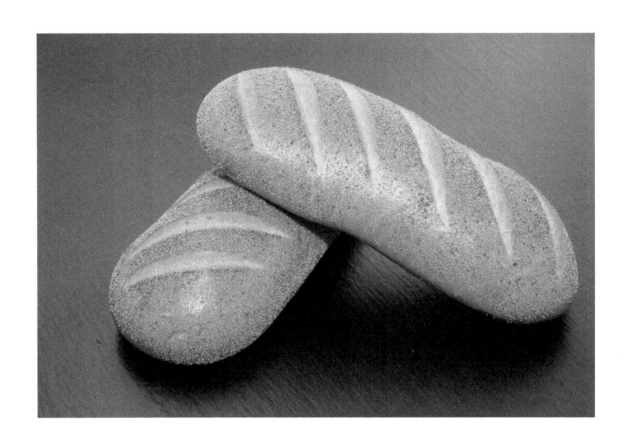

Keto Milk and Honey Breakfast Loaf

Nutrition Facts

Calories: 39

Calories from fat: 27

Total Fat: 3 g

Total Carbohydrates: 3 g

Net Carbohydrates: 3 g

Protein: 1 g

Preparation + Cook Time

Preparation Time: 2 hours

Cooking Time: 10 minutes

Total Time: 2 hours 10 minutes

Servings

18 slices

Ingredients

- 1 cup + 1 tbsp. almond milk, unsweetened

- 3 tbsps. honey

- 3 tbsps. melted butter

- 1 ½ tsp. salts

- 3 cups almond flour

- 2 tsps. active dry yeast

Directions

- Put all ingredients in the bread bucket as listed in the ingredient list.

- Select the BASIC cycle on your bread machine setting, close the lid then press START.

- Once the loaf is ready, remove from the machine and place in a cooling rack.

- Slice and serve with your favorite spread.

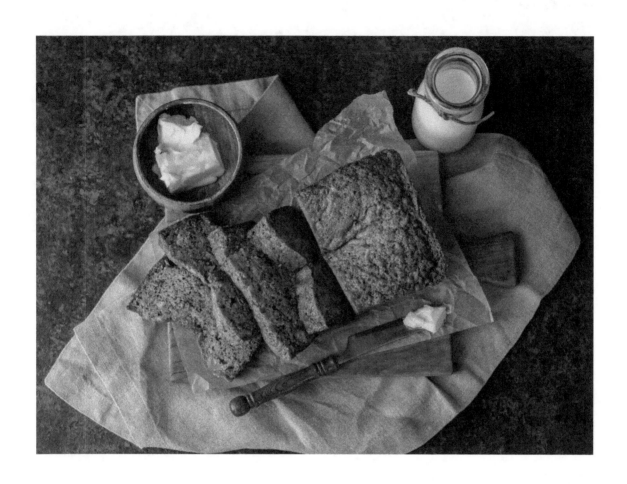

Keto Sweet Challah Bread

Nutrition Facts

Calories: 158

Calories from fat: 117

Total Fat: 13 g

Total Carbohydrates: 2 g

Net Carbohydrates: 2 g

Protein: 9 g

Preparation + Cook Time

Preparation Time: 20 minutes

Cooking Time: 3 hours

Total Time: 3 hours 20 minutes

Servings

20 slices

Ingredients

- 4 eggs

- 50 g sukrin plus

- 345 g cream cheese

- 60 g butter

- 60 g heavy cream

- 50 g vegetable oil

- 100 g unflavored whey protein

- 85 g protein whey vanilla

- ½ tsp. salt

- 3 g baking soda

- 12 g. baking powder

- 4 g xanthan

- ½ small lemon zest

- 30 g dried cranberries

Directions

- Place all ingredients on the bread machine pan except for lemon zest and cranberries.

- Select the SWEET BREAD cycle (or WHITE BREAD cycle) on the bread machine setting and light on the CRUST COLOR setting. Close the lid and press START.

- Just before the final rise, pause the bread machine and transfer the dough on a floured surface. Spread the dough and hand press the cranberries and lemon zest.

- Divide the dough into three equal parts. Roll each part of the dough to a 10-inch long rope. Lay all three ropes parallel to each other and braid together gently. Tuck the ends to form an oblong loaf. Brush the dough with egg white.

- Remove the kneading paddle of the bread machine before placing the dough back in the pan. Press START button again to resume the cycle.

- Once the cycle is finished, you can remove the challah and transfer it on a cooling rack.

- Slice and serve.

Keto Chocolate Loaf

Nutrition Facts

Calories: 95

Calories from fat: 80

Total Fat: 8 g

Total Carbohydrates: 3 g

Net Carbohydrates: 1 g

Protein: 4 g

Preparation + Cook Time

Preparation Time: 5 minutes

Cooking Time: 3 hours

Total Time: 3 hours 5 minutes

Servings

8 slices

Ingredients

- 1 cup almond milk, unsweetened

- 1 egg

- 1 egg yolk

- 3 tbsps. canola oil

- 1 tsp. vanilla extract

- 1 tsp. salt

- ½ cup brown sugar

- 1 tbsp. vital wheat gluten

- 1/3 cup cocoa

- 3 cups almond flour

- 2 ½ tsps. active dry yeast

Directions

- Put all ingredients on your bread machine bucket in the order of their appearance in the above list.

- Select BASIC cycle setting, and on the CRUST COLOR, select medium. Close the cover then press the START button.

- Wait for the cycle to finish before removing the loaf from the pan and transferring it on a cooling rack.

- Slice and serve with your favorite spread.

Keto Swiss cheese and Bacon Loaf

Nutrition Facts

Calories: 174

Calories from fat: 110

Total Fat: 12 g

Total Carbohydrates: 7 g

Net Carbohydrates: 6 g

Protein: 10 g

Preparation + Cook Time

Preparation Time: 20 minutes

Cooking Time: 2 hours 30 minutes

Total Time: 2 hours 50 minutes

Servings

10 slices

Ingredients

- 1 1/3 cups water

- 2 tbsps. vegetable oil

- 1 ¼ tsp. salt

- 2 tbsps. plus 1 ½ tsp. sugar

- 3 tbsps. dry milk, non-fat

- 4 cups almond flour

- 2 tsps. active dry yeast

- 2 cups Swiss cheese, shredded

- 3 tbsps. bacon bits

Directions

- Place all ingredients except the cheese and bacon in the order they appear on the ingredients list.

- Select BASIC cycle on your bread machine, close the cover and press START.

- When you hear a ping (fruit and nut signal), press pause and open the lid then add the cheese and bacon bits. Close the lid once more and press START to continue the cycle.

- When the cycle ends, transfer your loaf in a cooling rack.

- Slice and serve.

Keto Breakfast Muffin

Nutrition Facts

Calories: 124

Calories from fat: 90

Total Fat: 10

Total Carbohydrates: 6 g

Net Carbohydrates: 6 g

Protein: 2 g

Preparation + Cook Time

Preparation Time: 40 minutes

Cooking Time: 25 minutes

Total Time: 1 hour 5 minutes

Servings

12 muffin cups

Ingredients

- 1 cup almond milk

- 1 cup buttermilk

- 1 tsp. salt

- 4 tbsps. white sugar

- 2 eggs

- ½ cup melted butter

- 1 tbsp. baking powder

- 4 cups almond flour

Directions

- Place the all the ingredients onto the bread machine bucket in the order listed above.

- Select DOUGH cycle, close the lid, and press START button.

- When the bread machine pings, remove dough and transfer to a floured surface.

- Pour the muffin batter on a 12-cup muffin pan lined with muffin paper cups. Fill the cups 2/3 full then top with your favorite toppings.

- Pop in the oven and bake for 25 minutes or until tops are browned.

- Allow to cool down for around 5 minutes. Serve and enjoy.

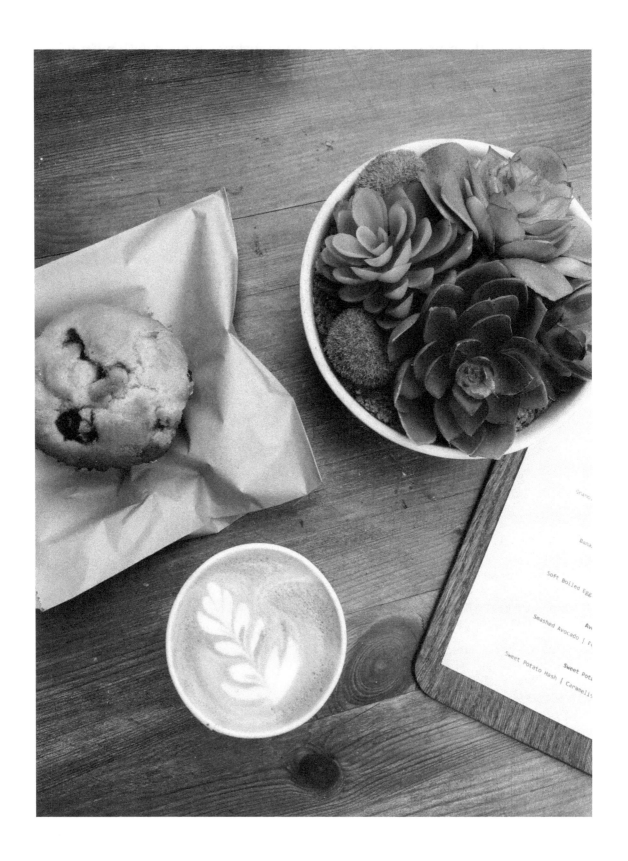

Keto Breakfast English Muffin

Nutrition Facts

Calories: 59

Calories from fat: 45

Total Fat: 5 g

Total Carbohydrates: 2 g

Net Carbohydrates: 2 g

Protein: 1 g

Preparation + Cook Time

Preparation Time: 3 hours 5 minutes

Cooking Time: 15 minutes

Total Time: 3 hours 20 minutes

Servings

10 pieces

Ingredients

- 1 cup almond milk, unsweetened

- 3 tbsps. butter, unsalted

- 1 egg

- ½ tsp. salt

- 2 tsp. white sugar

- 3 cups almond flour

- 1 ½ tsp. active dry yeast

Directions

- Put all the ingredients in the order listed above.

- Select DOUGH cycle setting from your bread machine. Close the lid, then press the START button.

- Once the cycle is finished, transfer the dough on a cornmeal sprinkled surface.

- Use your hand to pat and spread the dough into a ½-inch rectangle. Turn the dough so each side gets lightly dusted with cornmeal.

- Cut the dough into 10 rounds. Arrange each round on a baking sheet and let it rise for 20 to 30 minutes or until almost double in size.

- Heat a cast iron skillet over low flame and spray with cooking spray.

- Place the muffin on the heated skillet about 7 minutes each side until they turn golden brown.

Slice the muffin open and fill with your favorite jam and butter.

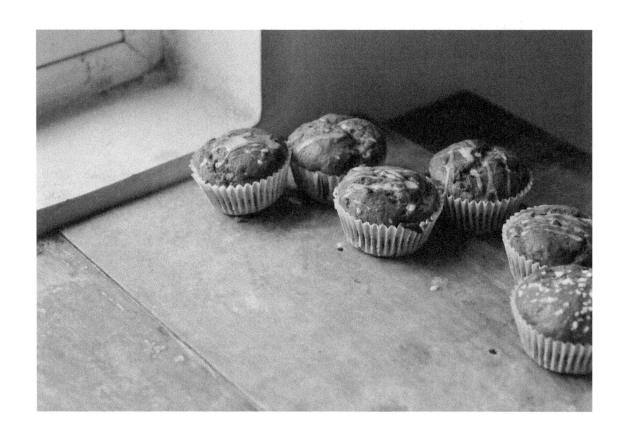

Keto Walnut Spice Bread

Nutrition Facts

Calories: 279

Calories from fat: 240

Total Fat: 26 g

Total Carbohydrates: 8 g

Net Carbohydrates: 6 g

Protein: 7 g

Preparation + Cook Time

Preparation Time: 10 minutes

Cooking Time: 2 hours

Total Time: 2 hours 10 minutes

Servings

10 slices

Ingredients

- 2 ¼ cup almond flour

- 1 tbsp. baking powder

- ¼ tsp. kosher salt

- 3 large eggs

- 1 ½ cup buttermilk

- 6 tbsp. canola oil

- 1 ½ cup brown sugar

- ½ tbsp. vanilla

- 1 ½ tsp. cinnamon

- 1/8 tsp. clove

- 1/8 tsp. allspice

- 1 cup rough chopped walnuts

Directions

- Place all the ingredients in your bread machine bucket except for the walnuts.

- Select the QUICK BREAD setting on your bread machine, close the cover then press START.

- Wait for the ping or the fruit and nut signal to open the lid and add the chopped walnuts. Close the lid again and press START to continue.

- When the cycle finishes, transfer the loaf to a wire rack and let it cool.

- Slice and serve with your favorite spread.

CHAPTER 4

Keto Bread Recipes for Lunch

Bread goes well with your salad and a great substitute if you want something light for lunch. You can eat breadsticks with your serve of keto pasta or grilled lemon chicken or how about grilled bacon and cheese sandwich with your favorite greens. Enjoy these mouthwatering bread recipes to satisfy your hunger.

Keto Flaxseed Honey Bread

Nutrition Facts

Calories: 96

Calories from fat: 36

Total Fat: 4 g

Total Carbohydrates: 5 g

Net Carbohydrates: 3 g

Protein: 8 g

Preparation + Cook Time

Preparation Time: 10 minutes

Cooking Time: 20 minutes

Total Time: 30 minutes

Servings

18 slices

Ingredients

- 1 cup warm water

- 2 small eggs, lightly beaten

- ½ cup oat fiber

- 2/3 cup flaxseed meal

- 1.25 cup vital wheat gluten

- 1 tsp. salt

- 4 tbsp. swerve powdered sweetener

- 1 tsp. honey

- ½ tsp. xanthan gum

- 2 tbsps. Butter, unsalted

- 1 tbsp. dry active yeast

Directions

- Pour the water on the bread bucket. e

- Add the eggs, honey, erythritol, salt, oat fiber, flaxseed meal, wheat gluten, and xanthan in this order. Add softened butter and yeast.

- Place back the bread bucket in your bread machine and close the lid. Select BASIC then select medium darkness on CRUST COLOR. Press START button and wait until the bread cooks.

- Cool bread on a cooling rack before slicing.

- Serve with grilled chicken or any of your favorite grilled meat. Note that nutrition info is only for the bread.

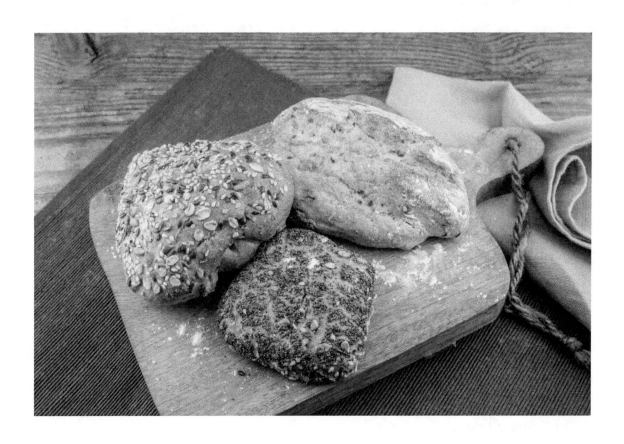

Keto Soft Pretzel Bread

Nutrition Facts

Calories: 217

Calories from fat: 162

Total Fat: 18 g

Total Carbohydrates: 3 g

Net Carbohydrates: 1 g

Protein: 11 g

Preparation + Cook Time

Preparation Time: 1 hours 45 minutes

Cooking Time: 15 minutes

Total Time: 2 hours

Servings

12 servings

Ingredients

- 3 cups mozzarella cheese

- 4 tbsps. Cream cheese

- 1 ½ cup almond flour

- 2 tsp. xanthan gum

- 2 small eggs

- 2 tsp. dried yeast

- 2 tbsps. Warm water

- 2 tbsps. Butter, melted and unsalted

- 1 tbsp. pretzel salt

Directions

- Melt the mozzarella and cream cheese in the microwave for 30 seconds.

- Dissolve the yeast in the warm water and 2 minutes to activate.

- In a bowl, combine all the dry ingredients and mix well.

- Using your bread bucket, pour the cheese mixture, the yeast mixture and the eggs.

- Add the dry ingredient mixture and 1 tbsp. of butter.

- Set the bread machine by selecting DOUGH, close the lid cover and press START button.

- After kneading, take out the dough from the bread bucket and cut into 12 balls.

- Preheat oven to 390 degrees F and prepare a lined cookie sheet.

- Roll out each ball into long sticks and twist into a pretzel shape and place on the cookie sheet.

- Brush the pretzel with the remaining 1 tbsp. butter and sprinkle with pretzel salt.

- Bake for around 15 minutes or until it turns golden brown.

- Serve with your favorite dip.

Keto Pepperoni Pizza

Nutrition Facts

Calories: 235

Calories from fat: 171

Total Fat: 19 g

Total Carbohydrates: 4 g

Net Carbohydrates: 2 g

Protein: 18 g

Preparation + Cook Time

Preparation Time: 1 hour 30 minutes

Cooking Time: 20 minutes

Total Time: 1 hour 55 minutes

Servings

8 servings

Ingredients

Crust

- 2 cups mozzarella cheese, shredded

- 2 tbsps. Cream cheese

- 1 egg

- ¾ cup almond flour

Toppings

- 1 ½ cup mozzarella cheese, shredded

- 1 tsp. Italian seasoning

- 1/3 cup Rao's Marinara sauce

- ¼ cup pepperoni, sliced

Directions

- To do the crust, melt the mozzarella and cream cheese in the microwave for 30 seconds. Transfer the cheese mixture in the bread bucket.

- Add the egg then add the almond flour. Close the lid of the bread machine.

- Turn the bread machine on by selecting DOUGH cycle and pressing the START button.

- Wait for the bread machine ping before taking out the dough.

- Preheat your oven to 425 degrees F. Spray your pizza pan with a non-stick spray and set aside.

- Place your dough between two parchment paper and flatten it using a rolling pan into 12-inch round diameter.

- Bake the dough for 10 minutes until lightly golden.

- Remove crust from oven and spread the marinara sauce over the crust.

- Sprinkle with mozzarella, and then arrange pepperoni on top.

- Allow to bake for about 10 minutes more.

- Cool down for about 5 minutes, then slice and serve.

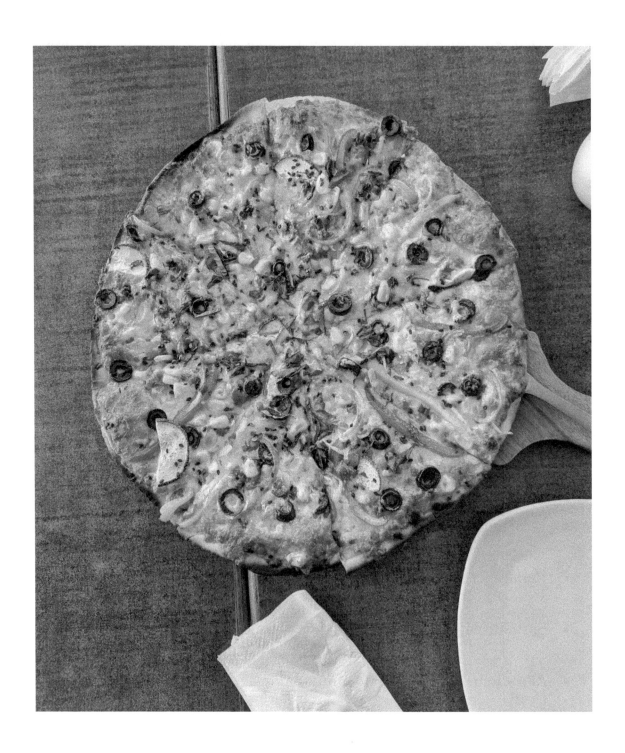

Keto Chicken and Ranch Pizza

Nutrition Facts

Calories: 311

Calories from fat: 225

Total Fat: 25 g

Total Carbohydrates: 6 g

Net Carbohydrates: 4 g

Protein: 16 g

Preparation + Cook Time

Preparation Time: 1 hour 40 minutes

Cooking Time: 15 minutes

Total Time: 1 hour 55 minutes

Servings

8 slices

Ingredients

Crust

- 2 cups mozzarella cheese, shredded

- 2 tbsps. Cream cheese

- 1 egg

- ¾ cup almond flour

- 1 tsp. salt

Ranch Sauce

- ½ cup mayonnaise

- ½ cup sour cream

- ¼ cup heavy cream

- 2 tbsps. White vinegar, distilled

- 2 cloves minced garlic

- 2 tbsps. Dill

- 1 tbsp. parsley

- 1 tsp. chives

- 1 tsp. onion powder

- 1 tsp. salt

Toppings

- 2 cups cheddar, shredded

- 1 cup grilled marinated chicken

- 6 strips bacon, fried and crumbled

- 2 tbsps. Chives, chopped

Directions

- Prepare the crust, melt the mozzarella and cream cheese in the microwave for 30 seconds. Transfer the cheese mixture in the bread bucket.

- Add the egg and salt, and then add the almond flour. Close the bread machine.

- Turn the bread machine on by selecting DOUGH cycle then press the START button.

- Wait for the bread machine to finish the dough cycle before taking out the dough.

- Prepare the ranch sauce by combining all ingredients together and whisking well.

- Preheat the oven at 425 degrees F and prepare a non-stick pizza pan. Set aside.

- Shape your dough into a 12-inch diameter round size. Slide it in the oven and bake for 12 minutes or until light golden.

- Spread 10 tablespoons of ranch over the crust and top with chicken, bacon and grated cheese. Pop back into the oven for 5 minutes or until cheese melts.

- Sprinkle with chives before slicing and serving.

Notes: Ranch recipe yields about 20 tablespoons.

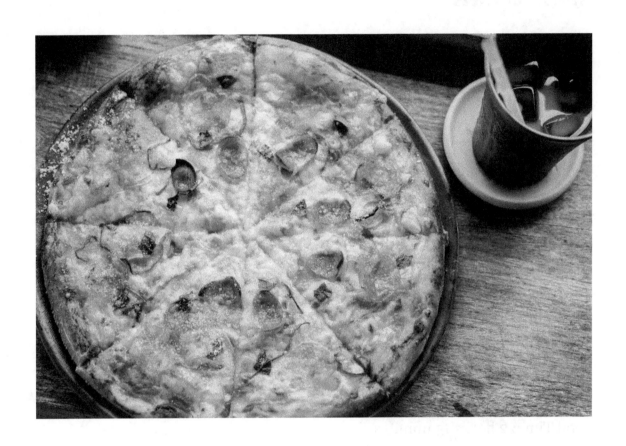

Keto Focaccia Squares

Nutrition Facts

Calories: 190

Calories from fat: 135

Total Fat: 15 g

Total Carbohydrates: 5 g

Net Carbohydrates: 3 g

Protein: 9 g

Preparation + Cook Time

Preparation Time: 2 hours

Cooking Time: 15 minutes

Total Time: 2 hours 15 minutes

Servings

9 squares

Ingredients

- 1 ½ cup mozzarella, shredded

- 1 oz. cream cheese, cubed

- 1 ½ cup almond flour, blanched

- 1 tbsp. baking powder

- 1 large egg, lightly beaten

Toppings

- 1 tbsp. rosemary leaves

- ½ tsp. coarse salt

Directions

- Melt the mozzarella and cream cheese in the microwave for 30 seconds. Stir then microwave for another 40 seconds.

- On you bread bucket, put the cheese, the egg, the almond flour, and the baking powder. Close the cover of the bread machine.

- Start your bread machine and set it to DOUGH cycle. Press the START button to start the cycle.

- Preheat your oven to 350 degrees Fahrenheit. Greased a 9-inch square pan.

- Take the dough out and press on a square baking pan. Put dimples on your dough using your fingers.

- Sprinkle your dough with rosemary leaves.

- Place in the oven and bake for 15 to 17 minutes or until golden brown.

- Cool the bread in a cooling rack for 15 minutes before cutting into nine squares.

- Serve.

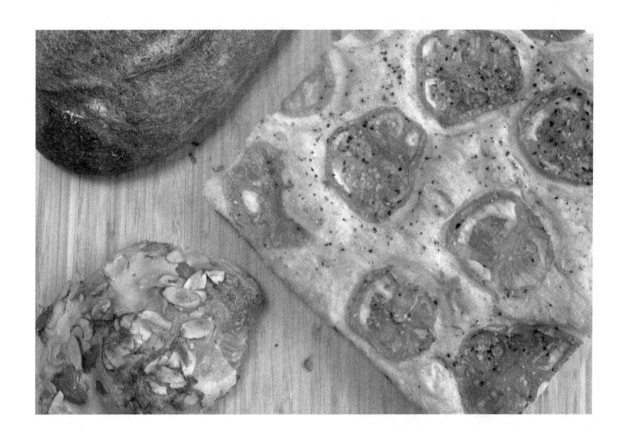

Keto Cajun Sandwich Loaf

Nutrition Facts

Calories: 35

Calories from fat: 9

Total Fat: 1 g

Total Carbohydrates: 5 g

Net Carbohydrates: 4 g

Protein: 1 g

Preparation + Cook Time

Preparation Time: 10 minutes

Cooking Time: 2 hours

Total Time: 2 hours 10 minutes

Servings

16 slices

Ingredients

- ½ cup water

- ¼ cup chopped onion

- ¼ cup chopped green bell peppers

- 2 tsp. fresh garlic, finely chopped

- 2 tsp. butter

- 2 cups almond flour

- 1 tbsp. sugar

- 1 tsp. Cajun seasoning

- ½ tsp. salt

- 1 tsp. active dry yeast

Directions

- Put all the ingredients in the loaf bucket of your bread machine then close the cover.

- Set your bread machine by selecting WHITE BREAD or BASIC cycle. Choose medium or dark color for CRUST COLOR setting. Press START.

- Once your loaf bread is finish, place it in a cooling rack.

- Slice and serve with ham and cheese to make a Cajun Ham and Cheese Sandwich.

Keto Flaxseed Sliced Bread

Nutrition Facts

Calories: 200

Calories from fat: 117

Total Fat: 13 g

Total Carbohydrates: 13 g

Net Carbohydrates: 3 g

Protein: 8 g

Preparation + Cook Time

Preparation Time: 5 minutes

Cooking Time: 3 hours

Total Time: 3 hours 5 minutes

Servings

15 slices

Ingredients

- 5 eggs

- ¼ cup coconut oil

- 2 tbsp. apple cider

- ½ tsp. salt

- 1 cup boiling water

- 1 tbsp. baking powder

- 2 tbsp. psyllium husk powder

- 2 cups flax seed flour

- ½ cup coconut flour

- ½ cup almond flour

- 2 tsp. dry active yeast

Directions

- Put all the ingredients in your bread machine bucket as listed above. Pull down the lid of the bread machine.

- Set your bread machine on BASIC cycle setting and select light on CRUST COLOR. Press the START button.

- Once the cycle is complete, take out the loaf from the bread machine and cool on a cooling rack.

- Slice and serve with cream cheese or any of your favorite spread.

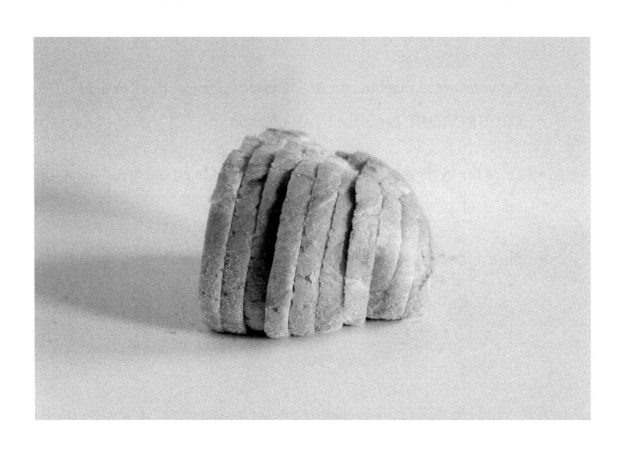

Keto Hamburger Buns

Nutrition Facts

Calories: 57

Calories from fat: 45

Total Fat: 5 g

Total Carbohydrates: 2 g

Net Carbohydrates: 2 g

Protein: 1 g

Preparation + Cook Time

Preparation Time: 2 hours 15 minutes

Cooking Time: 12 minutes

Total Time: 2 hours 27 minutes

Servings

8 buns

Ingredients

- 1 large egg

- ½ cup almond milk, unsweetened

- ¼ cup water

- 2 tbsp. unsalted butter

- 1 tbsp. granulated sugar

- ¾ tsp. salt

- 2 ½ cups almond flour

- 1 1/8 tsp. active dry yeast

Directions

- Put all ingredients in the order as listed above in your bread machine bucket.

- Close the lid. Start your machine by selecting DOUGH cycle then press START.

- Once the cycle is finished, transfer the dough on a floured surface. Cut the dough into 8-71 grams pieces. Form each piece into a ball and arranged on a greased lined baking sheet.

- Flatten each ball into 1/2-inch thick then cover. Leave the dough to rise until the size doubles or after 30-35 minutes.

- Preheat your oven at 400 degrees F. Pop the baking sheet into the oven and bake for 10-12 minutes or until golden brown.

- Remove from oven and let it cool in a wire rack.

- Serve with your Keto homemade burger or turkey slices.

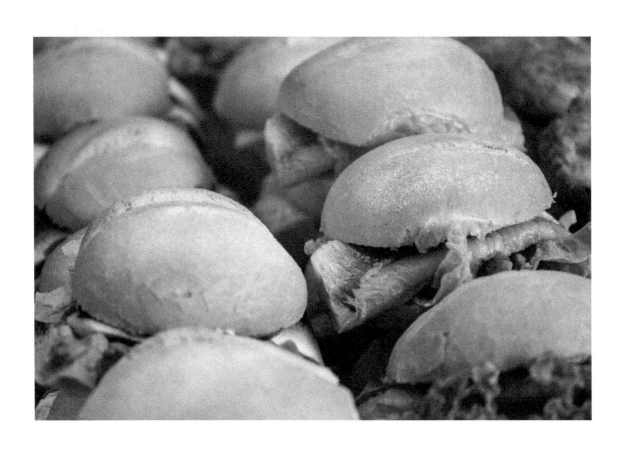

Keto German Franks Bun

Nutrition Facts

Calories: 49

Calories from fat: 45

Total Fat: 5 g

Total Carbohydrates: 1 g

Net Carbohydrates: 1 g

Protein:2 g

Preparation + Cook Time

Preparation Time: 2 hours

Cooking Time: 9 minutes

Total Time: 2 hours 9 minutes

Servings

10 buns

Ingredients

- 1 ¼ cup almond milk, unsweetened, warmed

- ¼ cup sugar, granulated

- 1 small egg

- 2 tbsps. butter

- ¾ tsp. salt

- 3 ¾ cups almond flour

- 1 ¼ tsps. active dry yeast

Directions

- Place all ingredients in your bread machine pan in the order listed above.

- Close the lid of your bread machine, select DOUGH cycle and press START.

- Once cycle is finish, transfer the dough into a floured surface. Cut the dough in 10 slices long.

- Flatten the dough into 5 x 4 inches. Then tightly roll the dough to form a cylindrical shape size of 5 x 1 inch. Cover and let it rise for an hour or until the dough size doubles.

- Preheat the oven at 350 degrees Fahrenheit. Arrange the dough in a greased baking sheet.

- Place the baking sheet in the oven and bake for 9 minutes or until golden brown.

- Cool then serve with your favorite franks.

Keto Beer Bread

Nutrition Facts

Calories: 118

Calories from fat: 90

Total Fat: 9

Total Carbohydrates: 3 g

Net Carbohydrates: 3 g

Protein: 6 g

Preparation + Cook Time

Preparation Time: 10 minutes

Cooking Time: 2 hours

Total Time: 2 hours 10 minutes

Servings

10 slices

Ingredients

- 10 oz. beer at room temperature

- 4 oz. American cheese, shredded

- 4 oz. Monterey Jack cheese, shredded

- 1 tbsp. sugar

- 1 ½ tsp. salt

- 1 tbsp. butter

- 3 cups almond flour

- 2.25 tsp. active dry yeast

Directions

- In a microwave, combine beer and American cheese and warm for 20 seconds.

- Transfer the beer mixture on the bread machine pan and add all the other ingredients as listed above.

- Close the bread machine lid and select WHITE BREAD setting (or BASIC setting) and press START button.

- When the cycle ends, cool the bread on a cooling rack.

- Slice and serve with a bowl of chili or beef stew.

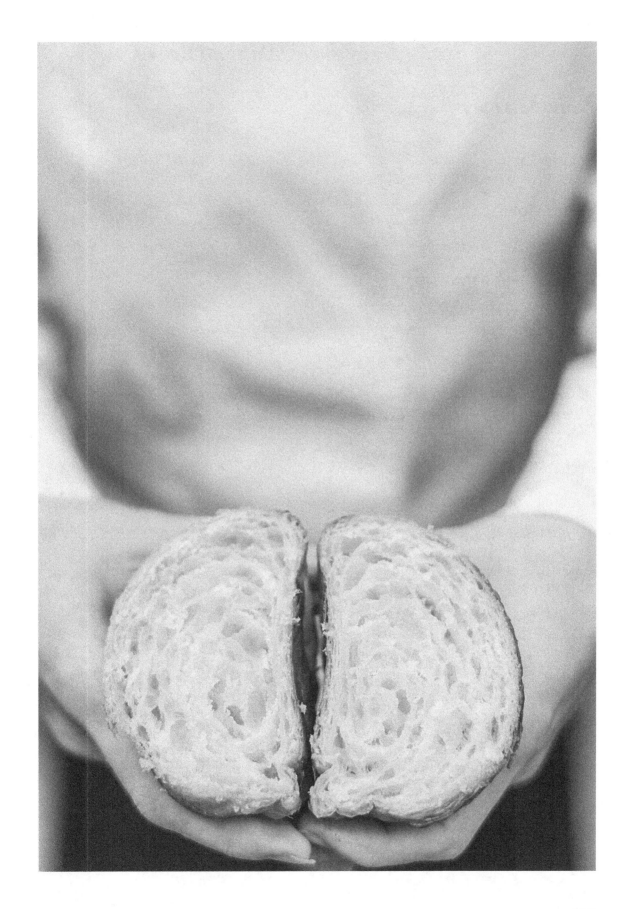

Keto Monterey Jack Jalapeno Bread

Nutrition Facts

Calories: 47

Calories from fat: 27

Total Fat: 3 g

Total Carbohydrates: 3 g

Net Carbohydrates: 2 g

Protein: 2 g

Preparation + Cook Time

Preparation Time: 15 minutes

Cooking Time: 2 hours

Total Time: 2 hours 15 minutes

Servings

12 slices

Ingredients

- 1 cup water

- 3 tbsps. non-fat milk

- 1 ½ tbsps. sugar

- 1 ½ tsp. salt

- 1 ½ tbsps. butter, cubed

- ¼ cup Monterey Jack cheese, shredded

- 1 small jalapeno pepper

- 3 cups almond flour

- 2 tsp. active dry yeast

Directions

- Remove the stem and seeds of the jalapeno and mince finely.

- Add the ingredients in the bread machine pan as listed above.

- Close the lid and select BASIC cycle and light or medium CRUST COLOR, then press START.

- Once the cycle ends, transfer the loaf in a cooling rack before slicing.

- Serve as a side dish for salad or your favorite main course.

Keto Pita Bread

Nutrition Facts

Calories: 37

Calories from fat: 27

Total Fat: 3 g

Total Carbohydrates: 2 g

Net Carbohydrates: 1 g

Protein: 1 g

Preparation + Cook Time

Preparation Time: 3 hours 5 minutes

Cooking Time: 15 minutes

Total Time: 3 hours 20 minutes

Servings

8 pieces

Ingredients

- 1 1/8 cups of warm water (110° F)

- 1 tsp. salt

- 1 tbsp. vegetable oil

- 1 ½ tsps. white sugar

- 3 cups almond flour

- 1 ½ tsp. active dry yeast

Directions

- Place all ingredients in the bread machine bucket.

- Pull down the cover and select DOUGH cycle setting before pressing START.

- When machine beeps, transfer the dough to a floured surface.

- Roll dough and stretch into a 12-inch long rope. Divide dough into 8 pieces then roll into a ball.

- Flatten each ball into a 6-7-inch circle. Cover and let it raise for 30 minutes.

- Preheat your oven at 500 degrees F. Place the pita bread on a wire rack and bake between 4-5 minutes or until it turns brown.

- Remove from the oven and immediately cover with a damp kitchen towel until it turns soft.

- Serve filled your favorite keto salad and meat.

Keto Rye Sandwich Bread

Nutrition Facts

Calories: 275

Calories from fat: 144

Total Fat: 16 g

Total Carbohydrates: 12

Net Carbohydrates: 8 g

Protein: 22 g

Preparation + Cook Time

Preparation Time: 10 minutes

Cooking Time: 3 hours

Total Time: 3 hours 10 minutes

Servings

12 slices

Ingredients

- 2 ¼ cups warm water

- 6 tbsps. melted butter, unsalted

- 2 tsps. white sugar

- 1 ½ tsp. salt

- 1 tbsp. baking powder

- ¼ tsp. ground ginger

- ¼ cup granulated swerve

- 2 cups vital wheat gluten

- 2 cups super fine almond flour

- ¼ cup dark rye flour

- 4.5 tsps. active dry yeast

- 1 tbsp. caraway seeds

Directions

- Place all ingredients in the bread machine bucket and close the lid.

- Select the WHOLE WHEAT cycle in your bread machine setting and choose light color on CRUST COLOR. Press START.

- When the cycle ends, remove the pan from the bread machine and transfer the loaf on a cooling rack.

- Slice and make a pastrami or Rueben sandwich to serve.

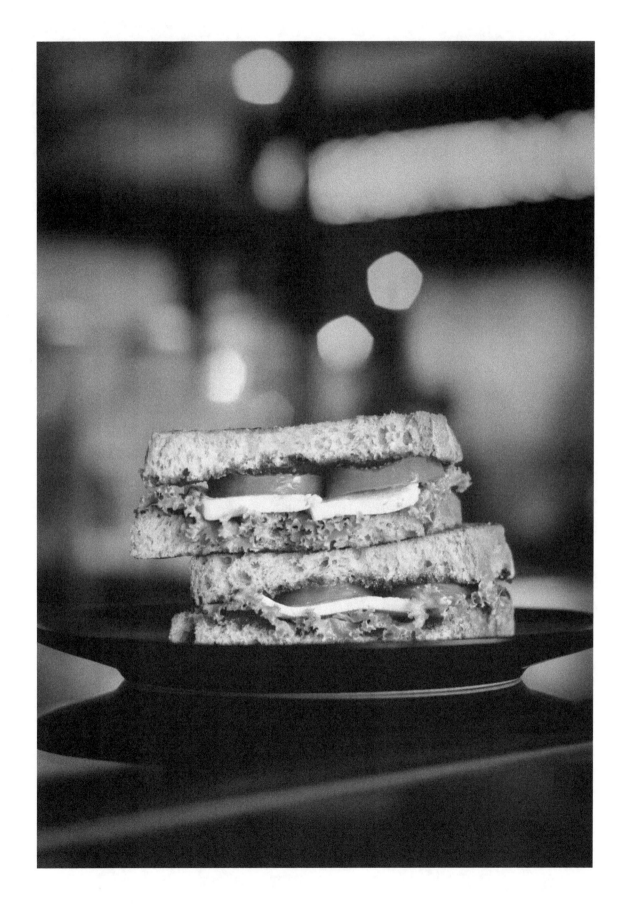

Keto Cheese Loaf Bread

Nutrition Facts

Calories: 90

Calories from fat: 70

Total Fat: 7 g

Total Carbohydrates: 4 g

Net Carbohydrates: 4 g

Protein: 4 g

Preparation + Cook Time

Preparation Time: 5 minutes

Cooking Time: 3 hours

Total Time: 3 hours 5 minutes

Servings

Ingredients

- 1 1/3 cup warm water

- 4 tbsps. non-fat powder milk

- 4 tbsps. melted butter, unsalted

- 2 tbsps. brown sugar

- 1 tbsp. Italian seasoning

- 2 tsps. salt

- 4 cups almond flour

- 1 ½ tsp. active dry yeast

- 1 cup shredded cheese

Directions

- Put all ingredients on the bread machine bucket in the order it is listed above. Do not include the shredded cheese.

- Close the cover then select the BASIC cycle setting and light color on CRUST COLOR setting then press START.

- Pause the bread machine after the final kneading and just before baking cycle. Open the lid and sprinkle the shredded cheese, then close the lid again and press START to continue.

- Once the cycle is complete, remove the bucket from the machine and transfer the loaf onto a cooling rack.

- Slice and serve plain or with spread.

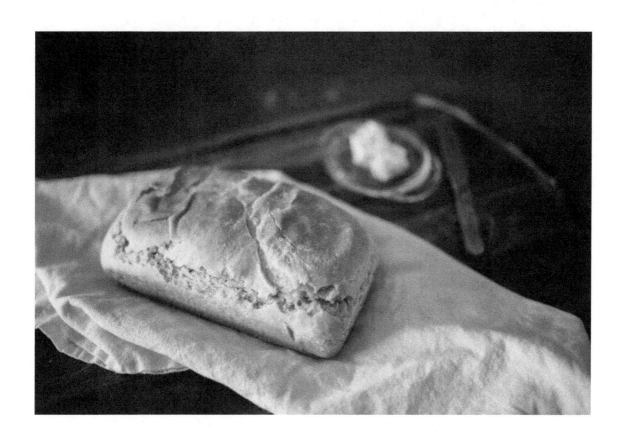

Keto Orange Cranberry Bread

Nutrition Facts

Calories: 141

Calories from fat: 110

Total Fat: 12 g

Total Carbohydrates: 5 g

Net Carbohydrates: 4 g

Protein: 4 g

Preparation + Cook Time

Preparation Time: 10 minutes

Cooking Time: 2 hours

Total Time: 2 hours 10 minutes

Servings

10 slices

Ingredients

- 2 ¼ cup almond flour

- 1 tbsp. baking powder

- ¼ tsp. kosher salt

- 3 large eggs

- 1 ½ cup buttermilk

- 6 tbsp. canola oil

- 1 ½ cup brown sugar

- ½ tbsp. vanilla

- ½ tsp. nutmeg

- ¾ tsp. orange zest

- 2 tbsp. orange juice, fresh

- 1 cup fresh cranberries, chopped

Directions

- Place all the ingredients in your bread machine bucket except for the cranberries.

- Close the bread machine before selecting QUICK BREAD setting on your bread machine then press START.

- Wait for the ping or the fruit and nut signal to open the lid and add the chopped cranberries. Close the lid again and press START to continue.

- When the cycle finishes, transfer the loaf to a wire rack and let it cool.

- Slice and serve with your favorite salad.

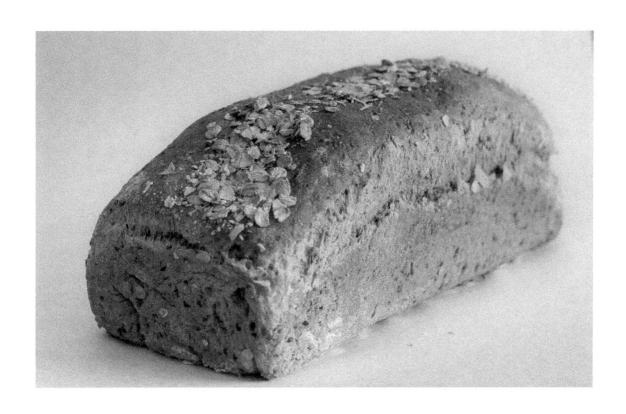

CHAPTER 5

Keto Bread Recipes for Dinner

At the end of the day, you are looking forward to a more relaxing night and you prefer something light to eat. Your mood calls for a fresh, light yet filling dinner to cap your day. Try these light, delicious and filling bread recipes.

Keto Dinner Rolls

Nutrition Facts

Calories: 38

Calories from fat: 27

Total Fat: 3 g

Total Carbohydrates: 2 g

Net Carbohydrates: 2 g

Protein: 1 g

Preparation + Cook Time

Preparation Time: 2 hours 5 min

Cooking Time: 15 minutes

Total Time: 2 hours 20 minutes

Servings

16 rolls

Ingredients

- 1 cup warm water

- 2 tbsp. margarine

- 1 tsp. salt

- 1 small egg, beaten

- ¼ cup sugar

- 3 cups almond flour

- 3 tsp. dry active yeast

- 3 tsp. melted butter for brushing

Directions

- Add in all ingredients in the bread bucket as listed in the ingredients. Place the bread bucket back in the bread machine. Close the lid cover.

- Turn the bread machine on then set it on DOUGH cycle and wait for the cycle to finish.

- Place the dough on a lightly floured table and shape into a long stick. Cut the dough into balls of 16 pieces and shape them into small buns. Place each bun in a non-stick pan leaving an inch between each bun.

- Brush the dough buns with melted butter and cover with a cling wrap then let it rise at warm temperature for 40 minutes.

- Preheat the oven at 375 degrees F. Bake the buns for 12 to 15 minutes.

- Serve warm.

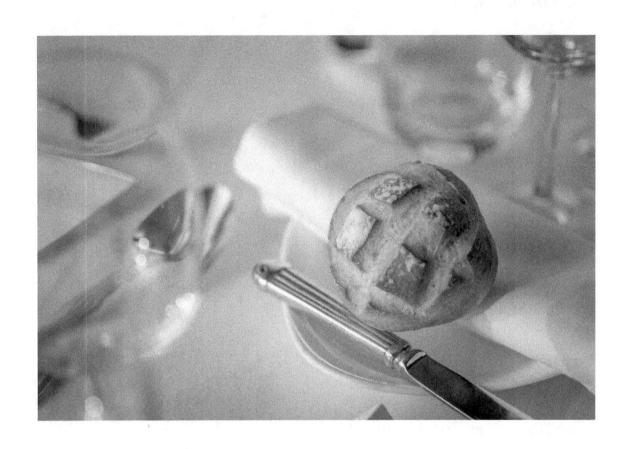

Keto BLT Fathead Pizza

Nutrition Facts

Calories: 317

Calories from fat: 234

Total Fat: 26 g

Total Carbohydrates: 6 g

Net Carbohydrates: 4 g

Protein: 15 g

Preparation + Cook Time

Preparation Time: 90 minutes

Cooking Time: 10 minutes

Total Time: 1 hour 40 minutes

Servings

6 slices

Ingredients

Crust

- 2 cups mozzarella cheese, shredded

- 2 tbsps. Cream cheese

- 1 egg

- ¾ cup almond flour

- 1 tsp. Italian seasoning

Toppings

- ¼ cup mayonnaise

- 1 ½ cup shredded lettuce

- ½ cup cherry tomatoes, cut in half

- 6 strip bacon, fried and diced

- 2 tbsps. Green onion, chopped

Directions

- To make the crust, melt the grated mozzarella and cream cheese in the microwave for 30 seconds. Transfer the cheese mixture in the bread bucket.

- Add the egg, salt, and Italian seasoning, and then add the almond flour. Lock in the bread bucket on the bread machine. Close the lid cover.

- Turn the bread machine on by selecting DOUGH cycle and press START.

- Wait for the bread machine to finish the dough cycle before taking out the dough.

- Preheat your oven at 425 degrees Fahrenheit.

- Roll out your dough into a round 12-inch diameter size and baked for 12 minutes on a non-stick pizza pan.

- Remove from oven and spread the mayonnaise before topping with lettuce, cherry tomatoes, bacon, and green onions.

- Slice and serve.

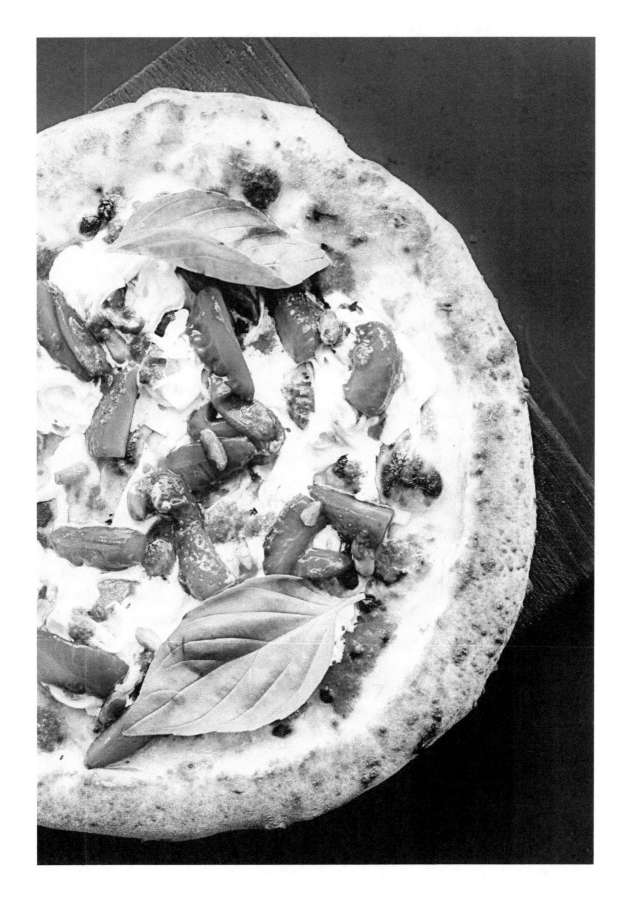

Keto Almond Pumpkin Quick Bread

Nutrition Facts

Calories: 70

Calories from fat: 60

Total Fat: 6 g

Total Carbohydrates: 2 g

Net Carbohydrates: 1 g

Protein: 1 g

Preparation + Cook Time

Preparation Time: 15 minutes

Cooking Time: 60 minutes

Total Time: 1 hour 15 minutes

Servings

16 slices

Ingredients

- 1/3 cup vegetable oil

- 3 large eggs

- 1 ½ cup pumpkin puree, canned

- 1 cup granulated sugar

- 1 ½ tsp. baking powder

- ½ tsp. baking soda

- ¼ tsp. salt

- ¾ tsp. ground cinnamon

- ¼ tsp. ground nutmeg

- ¼ tsp. ground ginger

- 3 cups almond flour

- ½ cup chopped pecans

Directions

- Spray your bread machine pan with cooking spray.

- In a bowl, mix all the wet ingredients until blended. Add all the dry ingredients except pecans until mixed.

- Pour the batter onto your bread machine pan and place it back inside the bread machine. Close the cover securely.

- Turn on the bread machine and select QUICK BREAD cycle then press START.

- When your bread machine pings, pause and open the lid then add the chopped pecans. Then close the lid and press START to let the cycle continue.

- Once cycle is finished, loosen the loaf from the pan and transfer to a cooling rack.

- Slice and serve with your favorite keto soup.

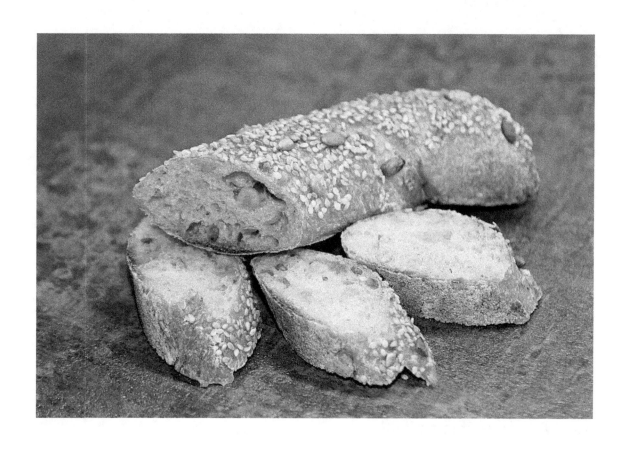

Keto Basil Parmesan Slices

Nutrition Facts

Calories: 40

Calories from fat: 27

Total Fat: 3 g

Total Carbohydrates: 3 g

Net Carbohydrates: 3 g

Protein: 1 g

Preparation + Cook Time

Preparation Time: 10 minutes

Cooking Time: 2 hours

Total Time: 2 hours 10 minutes

Servings

16 slices

Ingredients

- 1 cup water

- ½ cup parmesan cheese, grated

- 3 tbsps. sugar

- 1 tbsp. dried basil

- 1 ½ tbsps. olive oil

- 1 tsp. salt

- 3 cups almond flour

- 2 tsps. active dry yeast

Directions

- Place all the ingredients in your bread machine pan according the list stated in the ingredients list.

- Close the lid then set the bread machine on BASIC cycle and press START.

- Once cycle is done, move loaf to a cooling rack.

- Slice and serve as side dish for your soup or main course.

Keto Slider Rolls

Nutrition Facts

Calories: 51

Calories from fat: 36

Total Fat: 4 g

Total Carbohydrates: 3 g

Net Carbohydrates: 2 g

Protein: 1 g

Preparation + Cook Time

Preparation Time: 80 minutes

Cooking Time: 25 minutes

Total Time: 1 hour 45 minutes

Servings

18 rolls

Ingredients

- ½ cup warm water (110 degrees F)

- 2/3 cup almond milk, unsweetened

- 1 large egg

- 3 tbsps. melted butter, unsalted

- 2 tbsps. + 1.5 tsp. sugar

- 1.25 tsp. salt

- 3 cups almond flour

- 2.25 tsp. active dry yeast

Egg wash

- 1 large egg white

- 1 tbsp. water

- ¼ cup sesame seeds

Directions

- Gather all ingredients and put in the bread machine pan in order of appearance in the ingredients list.

- Close the bread machine then set the bread machine on DOUGH cycle and press START button.

- After the cycle ends, transfer the dough in a floured surface and knead 6 to 8 times before resting for 10 minutes in a rectangular.

- Cut into 18 pieces about 1.5 oz. to 1.75 oz. each piece.

- Shape each piece in a ball and arrange 3 to 4 inches apart on a non-stick baking sheet. Flatten each ball slightly with your hand.

- Cover the buns and let it rise for about 30 minutes.

- Preheat your oven to 375 degrees F.

- Prepare the egg wash by whisking egg white and water until blended.

- Before popping in the oven, brush each bun with the egg wash and sprinkle with sesame seeds.

- Bake for about 15 to 18 minutes or until it turns golden brown.

- Cool the buns in a cooling rack and split apart.

- Serve with pulled pork, shredded beef or any of your favorite fillings.

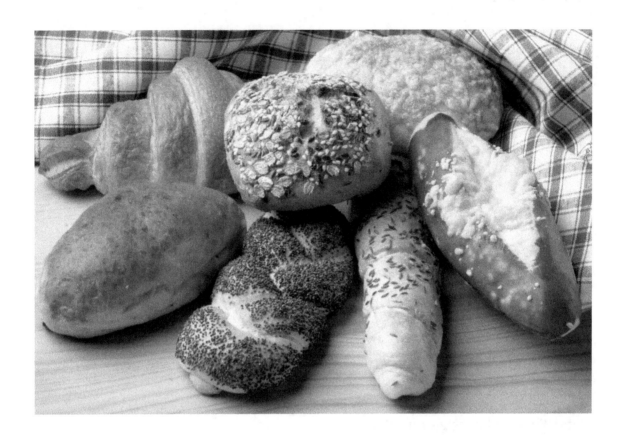

Keto Onion Bread

Nutrition Facts

Calories: 62

Calories from fat: 36

Total Fat: 4 g

Total Carbohydrates: 5 g

Net Carbohydrates: 4 g

Protein: 2 g

Preparation + Cook Time

Preparation Time: 25 minutes

Cooking Time: 2 hours

Total Time: 2 hours 25 minutes

Servings

12 slices

Ingredients

- 1 ½ cups water

- 2 tbsp. + 2 tsp butter, unsalted

- 1 ½ tsp. salt

- 1 tbsp. + 1 tsp. sugar

- 2 tbsp. + 2 tsp. non-fat dry milk

- 4 cups almond flour

- 2 tsp. active dry yeast

- 4 tbsps. dry onion soup mix

Directions

- Add all ingredients except dry onion mix in the bread machine pan according to the list above.

- Close the lid cover. Select BASIC cycle on your bread machine and then press START.

- Your machine will ping after around 30 to 40 minutes. This is your signal to add whatever fruit, nut or flavoring you wish to add to your dough. Pause your bread machine and add the dry onion soup mix.

- Press START again and allow the cycle to continue.

- Once your loaf is finish, transfer it to a cooling rack.

- Slice and serve with cream cheese or butter or as a soup side dish.

Keto Sundried Tomato Quick Bread

Nutrition Facts

Calories: 144

Calories from fat: 110

Total Fat: 12 g

Total Carbohydrates: 6 g

Net Carbohydrates: 5 g

Protein: 4 g

Preparation + Cook Time

Preparation Time: 10 minutes

Cooking Time: 2 hours

Total Time: 2 hours 10 minutes

Servings

10 slices

Ingredients

- 2 ¼ cup almond flour

- 1 tbsp. baking powder

- 1 tsp. kosher salt

- 3 large eggs

- 1 ½ cup buttermilk

- 6 tbsp. canola oil

- 1 tbsp. dried basil

- 1 cup sundried tomato roughly chopped

Directions

- Place all the ingredients in your bread machine bucket except for basil and sundried tomato.

- Secure the lid cover. Select the QUICK BREAD setting on your bread machine then press START.

- Wait for the ping or the fruit and nut signal to open the lid and add the basil and sundried tomato. Close the lid again and press START to continue.

- When the cycle finishes, transfer the loaf to a wire rack and let it cool.

- Slice and serve.

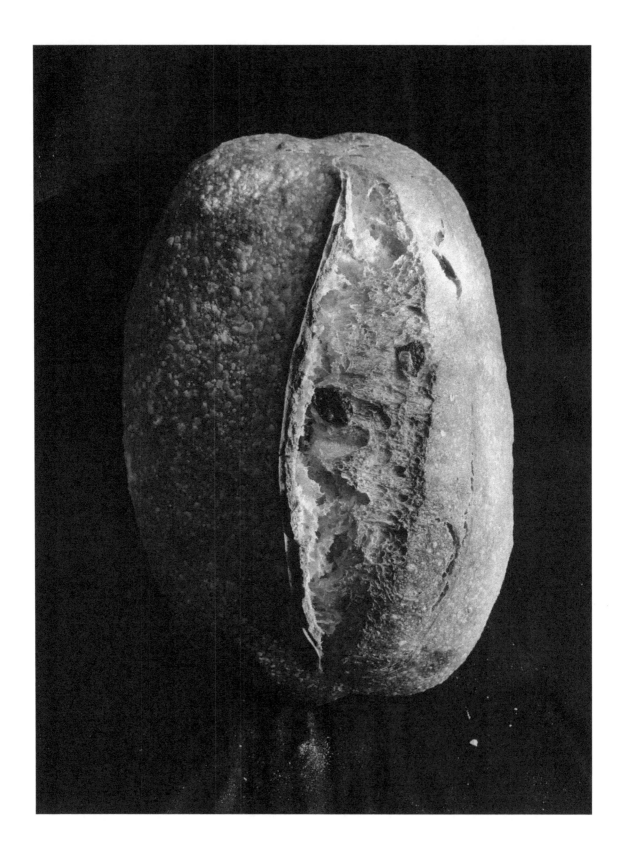

Keto Cheddar Bacon and Chive Bread

Nutrition Facts

Calories: 164

Calories from fat: 140

Total Fat: 15 g

Total Carbohydrates: 3 g

Net Carbohydrates: 3 g

Protein: 6 g

Preparation + Cook Time

Preparation Time: 10 minutes

Cooking Time: 2 hours

Total Time: 2 hours 10 minutes

Servings

10 slices

Ingredients

- 2 ¼ cup almond flour

- 1 tbsp. baking powder

- 1 tsp. kosher salt

- 3 large eggs

- 1 ½ cup buttermilk

- 6 tbsp. canola oil

- 3 tbsp. finely chopped chives

- 1 cup shredded cheddar sharp cheese

- 6 strips bacon cook and crumbled

Directions

- Place all the ingredients in your bread machine bucket pan except for bacon.

- Close the cover. Select the QUICK BREAD setting on your bread machine then press START.

- Wait for the fruit and nut signal. Pause and open the lid and add the bacon. Close the lid again and press START to continue.

- When the cycle finishes, transfer the loaf to a wire rack and let it cool.

- Slice and serve.

Keto Tortilla Wraps

Nutrition Facts

Calories: 170

Calories from fat: 117

Total Fat: 13 g

Total Carbohydrates: 9 g

Net Carbohydrates: 1 g

Protein: 5 g

Preparation + Cook Time

Preparation Time: 40 minutes

Cooking Time: 10 minutes

Total Time: 50 minutes

Servings

6 servings

Ingredients

- 1 cup golden flaxseed meal

- 2 tbsps. coconut flour

- ½ tsp xanthan gum

- ½ tsp. salt

- 1 tbsp. butter

- 1 cup warm water

Directions

- Add all ingredients in your bread machine. Close the lid cover.

- Select DOUGH cycle and press START.

- Once the cycle is finish, remove the dough and transfer to a lightly floured working table.

- Divide the dough to equal chunks. Roll out the dough into a thin shape.

- On a skillet over low heat, cook the tortilla for 1-2 minutes each tortilla. Remove from the skillet and cover with a towel. The tortillas should be soft and not stiff.

- Serve with your favorite filling.

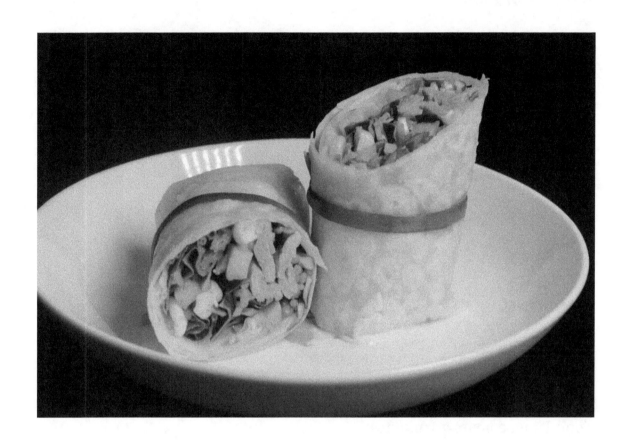

Keto Southern Biscuit

Nutrition Facts

Calories: 112

Calories from fat: 90

Total Fat: 9 g

Total Carbohydrates: 5 g

Net Carbohydrates: 4 g

Protein: 4 g

Preparation + Cook Time

Preparation Time: 2 hours 15 minutes

Cooking Time: 15 minutes

Total Time: 2 hours 30 minutes

Servings

10 biscuits

Ingredients

- 2/3 cup milk

- 2 large eggs, lightly beaten

- 1/3 cup butter, unsalted and softened

- 1 tbsp. honey

- 1 ¼ tsp. salt

- 3 ½ cups almond flour

- 3 tsp. active dry yeast

Directions

- Place all the ingredients according to the list arrangement above. Close the bread machine lid.

- On your bread machine, select DOUGH cycle then press the START button.

- Once the cycle ends, remove the dough and transfer to a floured working table. Roll out the dough until it is ½-inch thick.

- Cut into 10 sizes and arrange on a greased baking sheet. Let it rise for an hour.

- Preheat your oven to 425 degrees F.

- Pop the baking sheet into the oven and bake for 15 minutes or until lightly golden.

- Serve with your favorite soup or fill with your favorite meat filling.

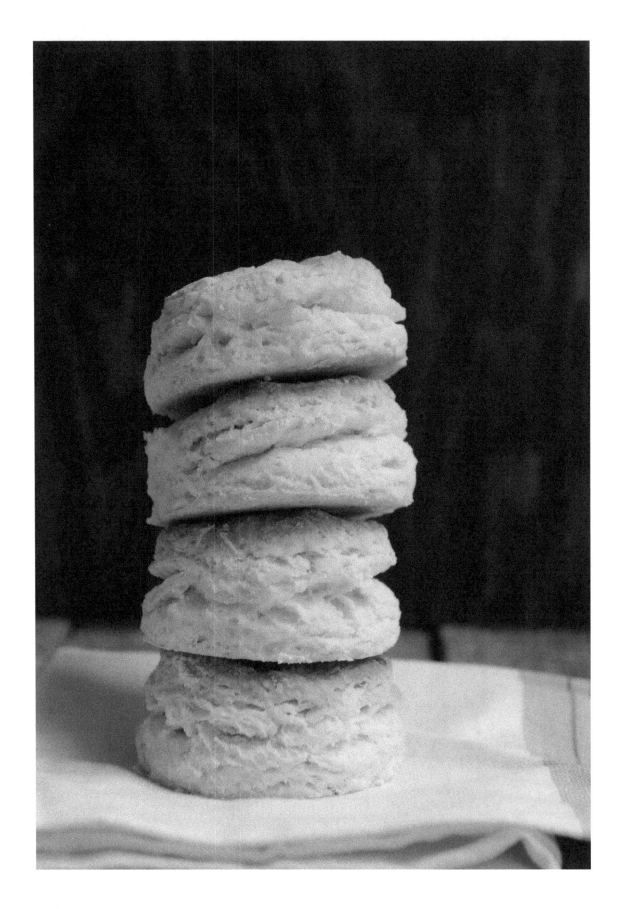

CONCLUSION

I'd like to thank you and congratulate you for transiting my lines from start to finish.

I hope this book was able to help you understand the Keto Diet better. I hope you also learned some tricks on how to maintain being in ketosis and guide you on what to do in situations that you would kick you out of the ketogenic stage.

I also hope that the recipes shared in this book have helped you in adding new food that you can eat while in Keto. You can use the bread recipes included in this book interchangeably for breakfast, lunch and dinner and you can prepare them easily with the use of a bread machine.

The next step is making these bread recipes part of your keto meal plan. It is easy to prepare and a meal alternative, especially for people on the go.

I wish you the best of luck!

BONUS CONTENT

MEAL PREP CHAPTER **2**

On Mindful Eating and Curbing Hunger

Switching to a healthier lifestyle, especially after you've been used to doing things a way for so long will take some adjustment. There will be challenges and you might find yourself falling behind at certain points—understand that this is totally fine. What matters is that you get back on track, exert a bit more effort, and make some necessary changes that will support the kind of life you want to have.

When it comes to eating healthier, it's more than just selecting the right food and doing portion control. Your overall mental approach matters just as much and being mindful about how you do things can really help make things easier. With that said, here are a few Do's and Don'ts to keep in mind.

The Do's

1.   Do start with your shopping list.

Always take your time and make sure you feel focused when writing your list. Mindfulness is key when it comes to creating the right grocery list that will benefit your goals. Think about how you've been feeling lately—what does your body require now? With that in mind, start putting together your choices and edit it as you go.

2.   Do savor your meals.

Here's the thing, most people rush through their meals because of various reasons. Some may not have a lot of time to spare, whilst there are those who want to use that time for something else "more important". However, it is important to relish your food; take the time to enjoy its flavor, its aroma, and chew properly. Eating mindfully also makes you feel sated for a longer period.

3.   Do the "mouth full, hands empty" mantra.

This means that you should set your cutlery down in between mouthfuls of food. Quite similar to the previous tip, this is meant to help slow you're eating and enable you to better appreciate your food. Not only that, doing this can actually help increase the response of your gut peptides. You'll feel full for longer and keep you from overeating.

4. Always wait a minute or two before going back for seconds.

This allows the food you just ate to settle down and give you enough time to think if you really want more. Most people have a tendency to immediately go for seconds right after eating, especially if the food is something they really like. However, this often leads to them feeling too full and bloated. So, take your time after finishing your plate. Have some water or a sip of tea, then decide if you really need to refill your plate.

5. Do keep your bigger serving bowls of food off the table and out of sight.

This is to serve the previous step's purpose. If you cannot immediately see or reach the food, you won't be able to refill your plate quickly. It also keeps you from craving more just because you keep seeing food. As you may or may not know, just the mere visual of delicious food can make us overeat. If we can see it and smell even while eating, we're bound to grab more servings.

The Don'ts

6. Don't eat while you're distracted by something.

A lot of us fall into the trap of multi-tasking; in this case, eating whilst doing something else. Maybe you do it while you're watching TV, while you're working, or while you're moving from one place to the next. Sure, it feels good to be accomplishing a lot of things at the same time, but did you know that this can be detrimental to your fitness goals? By doing this, you're likelier to overeat or end up snacking again later. This is because your brain isn't fully processing the fact that you're eating.

So next time, give yourself an hour or 30 minutes to eat your meals.

7.   Don't drink too much alcohol before you begin eating.

Aside from its calorie content, research has shown that people who drink more before eating are more prone to cheating on their diets. Alcohol is also known to stimulate are appetites, making it harder for us to say no to food we cannot have.

8.   Don't eat when you're feeling stressed.

A lot of us tend to "eat our feelings" as a means of relieving stress or any emotional distress we may be experiencing. Whilst this does seem to work, it can also cause us to overeat and feel guilty later on. Instead of turning to food during stressful moments, try mindfulness meditation instead. This will help turn our attention away from what we're craving (usually very indulgent food items) and is also a healthier alternative to stress eating.

9.   Don't forego your diet just because you're eating out.

As we've already established, there are ways of still following your diet even when you're out with friends. Remember, people also tend to eat more when they're in social settings or surrounded by friends. Don't stress yourself out when the menu for an event or a restaurant does not fit into your WW freestyle diet. Where you might not be able to be pickier of what you eat, you can always opt for portion sizes.

Eating mindfully is one thing, but the real challenge often happens when you're trying to beat hunger. It can make just about anyone restless and even cranky—everyone's familiar with this. Here are a few do's and don'ts to keep in mind when it comes to curbing your hunger:

The Do's

10.   Do your best to always get enough sleep.

Not getting enough sleep affects the balance of your hormones related to the appetite. Research shows that people who have had less than 5 hours of sleep experienced an increase in the ghrelin levels in their body. This is the hormone which actually triggers appetite and decreases leptin levels. Leptin is the hormone that signals our brain when we've had enough food.

11.   Do a bit of cardio after eating.

Doing this has a positive effect on our satiety hormones, helping promote a longer feeling of satiety. Research also proves that doing moderate-intensity exercises can curb feelings of hunger. It is also an effective form of distraction, keeping you from unintentionally eating or snacking.

When you start feeling the need to snack, try going for a walk instead. After you get back from it, you're bound to feel less inclined to grab a bag of chips or snack on your favorite treats. Note that the brain actually enjoys when we form new habits so do try and focus on making healthier ones, instead of trying to break your current bad habits. You'll eventually replace them when the good habits stick.

12.   Do have a hearty breakfast.

Breakfast is important—essential to our day. Having a hearty one provides our body with the ample fuel it needs to give you a head start on the day. People who begin their day with a protein-rich breakfast are less likely to begin craving snacks halfway through their morning. It also keeps you from overeating when lunchtime comes around, effectively preventing body fat gain and enabling you to manage your hunger better.

The Don'ts

13.   Don't eat too many fatty foods.

Having too much dietary fat in your daily meals can actually trigger ghrelin, the hunger hormone. Basically, the fattier the food you eat is, the greater your appetite for it would become. Just think back to all the times you've eaten food like French fries, pizzas, steaks, and so on—it's usually really hard to stop, right? Therefore.

Another thing to pay attention to is your low-fat food's total energy content. These types of food is likely to contain great amounts of sugar to compensate for any flavor that's lost due to the low-fat content.

14.   Don't deprive yourself of your favorite foods.

It's totally okay to enjoy the foods you love, but make sure you do so moderately. Doing so actually helps you deal with cravings better and makes you feel less guilty about having them as well. Banning a food only serves to increase your craving for it so don't be afraid to have your favorites whenever you really feel like them.

Printed in the USA
CPSIA information can be obtained
at www.ICGtesting.com
LVHW082255140524
780324LV00038B/1372